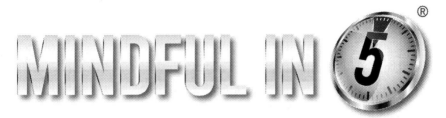

MINDFUL IN 5

Meditations for People *with* No Time

SPIWE JEFFERSON, CMP, JD

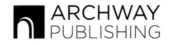

ARCHWAY
PUBLISHING

Archway Publishing books may be ordered through booksellers or by contacting:

Archway Publishing
1663 Liberty Drive
Bloomington, IN 47403
www.archwaypublishing.com
844-669-3957

ISBN: 978-1-6657-2054-0 (sc)
ISBN: 978-1-6657-2052-6 (hc)
ISBN: 978-1-6657-2053-3 (e)

Library of Congress Control Number: 2022911562

Print information available on the last page.

Archway Publishing rev. date: 6/23/2022

CONTENTS

DAWN

ACKNOWLEDGMENTS

Papa, thank you for this life.

To Mama, the late Professor Rosemary Moyana PhD, pro vice chancellor, University of Zimbabwe, thank you for fathomless love.

To Dad, His Excellency, the late Dr. Henry V. Moyana, Zimbabwean Ambassador to Egypt, thank you for your example of tireless industry.

To super-smart Jamie, songstress Moyana Olivia, brave Bernie, and cool Jet, I love you. Always shine on!

To TJ, thank you for selfless devotion to God and our family.

Nyasha Moyana and the Jefferson, Moyana, Manase, and Mugugu clans, thank you for always being there.

To Jerry W. Blackwell, thank you for introducing me to this path. To Mr. Bill Fridge, Master, the leaders, and devotees of Self-Realization Fellowship (SRF), the Mindfulness-Based Stress Reduction (MBSR) Institute, and the Life Success Academy, thank you for growing my practice.

To Renée Aikens, Brent Bauer, Jasmine Brett Stringer, Renée Clippert, Leslie Davis Niemoeller, Sonya Harris, Bridgette Herndon, Melanie Jones, Ben Omorogbe, Jaymie Turner, my beta readers, the Bench & Bar Book Club, CarMoBarSpi, My Sister's Keeper, Sisters Circle, my amazing neighbor friends, and my Chicago crew, thank you for boundless friendship and support.

WHY I WROTE THIS BOOK

I am surrounded by powerful people: powerhouse professionals, devoted parents, and successful executives. These people look like they have it all. But in quiet moments of intimate conversation, they say things like:

"Why do I still feel like I'm not good enough?"
"I thought achieving this level of success in my career would make me happy."
"Is this all there is?"

We are surrounded by fear, division, and the perception of scarcity. Technology keeps us connected more than ever, yet depression and loneliness are on the rise. And more people seem to have trouble turning off their minds or sleeping. With every complaint I thought, *I have a suggestion for that.*

My Wilderness Journey

Years ago, my life was in turmoil. I was getting divorced, and at stake was everything I had counted on: my marriage, children, home, friends, finances, and future plans. Some psychologists say death and divorce are among the worst experiences we can encounter. My father, who I loved and respected, had a heart attack and passed away three months after my divorce was final. For years I felt adrift in a wilderness with no light on the horizon. How I found my way through that dark and desolate time is reflected in the pages of this book.

My Way Back on the Mindfulness Meditation Path

In 2005 a friend introduced me to meditation. A devoted lover of God, I have long been a student of the Bible. But while Jesus taught us how to pray, and the Bible instructs us to meditate, it provides no step-by-step guide to meditation.

Thus began my journey of meditative learning. I studied formal meditation lessons; read numerous books on mindfulness and meditation; and attended meditation sessions, services, conferences, and retreats. I practiced using various tools and techniques under the guidance of yogis and experts. I became a certified mindfulness practitioner, and because mindfulness meditation is a path and not a destination, I continue to be a student of devotional, self-help, and inspirational books on how to weather life's challenges.

How Mindfulness Changed My Life

It didn't happen in a day, a week, or a month. But over time, I recovered from the emotional devastation of my personal losses and came into a new realm of ever-new joy, love, and peace. Mindfulness meditation accelerated that process and gave birth to a much stronger, calmer, and more centered self. Before, I was a reed tossed about by the winds of emotional and daily upheaval. Now I'm an oak tree, firm and stable even when the howling gales of change and calamity arise. It doesn't exempt me from the ups and downs of life, but it does allow me to stand strong through them from an emotional and psychological place of equanimity and power.

What Mindfulness Can Do for You

This power is within you, too, and this book will help you to unleash it. I wrote this book because I long to share the inner peace and strength I have found to weather life's challenges.

Mindfulness meditation will not solve your problems. But with consistent practice, it will improve your outlook, attitude, and overall quality of life. It will unlock and unleash your inner strength, allowing you to overcome the challenges of daily life with a deeper calm and an unflappable focus.

Whether you are a novice who has never meditated before or a seasoned yogi with years of practice, this book provides topics you can use in any season of life. I extend joy and peace to you as you explore your life at a deeper level by walking through the pages of this book.

May you harness the power of mindfulness to live and work to your highest and best purpose each day. Win the game of life no matter what challenges you face.

HOW TO USE THIS BOOK

You don't have to read this book in sequence. Choose your own adventure from three seasons, fifty-two weeks, five minutes of meditation per day, five reflections per week.

Regardless of how new or mature you are on the mindfulness meditation path, take a gander through the "Practice" section. After "Practice," three parts follow: "Dark," "Dawn," and "Day." Here we meet four strangers who become friends during a year of attending a support group together. Their journey through the seasons illustrates their individual struggles and how they harness the power of mindfulness to face the ups and downs of each day.

Because it can be challenging to sit still even for five minutes at a time, use the topics to center your thoughts. On any given day, however, feel free to veer off topic and focus on any issue relevant to you in the moment.

Three Seasons

While weather seasons are not the same around the world, every day can be divided into the same three parts: dark, dawn, and day. In this book, each season represents a different time in your life, or simply how you feel from one day to the next.

You may feel that what I am calling "seasons" are out of order; after all, shouldn't they be organized in the same progression as during a regular day—dawn, day, dark? No. The order is intentional. Most people become reflective and seek answers when facing difficulties, hence the book begins with dark. Once you make it through this season, you then encounter dawn, a season of new possibilities that carries you into the bright sun of day.

Pegin by reading the "Practice" chapters. Journey into mindfulness meditation with two friends as one, Akar, struggles with many challenges you might face in getting started on your mindfulness meditation journey. Chantelle is a mindful ninja; she cheers you on and provides suggestions to help you troubleshoot your practice. And she shows you what life can look like when you're on your mindfulness game.

 Dark: In this season you encounter the worst emotional and psychological pain of your life. It could be triggered by a job loss, someone's death, a significant breakup, a pandemic, a terrible medical diagnosis, or physical or psychological trauma. You may question yourself, your life, and everything you thought was true. This is when it is most critical to take time and set your intentions and mental framework each day.

 **Dawn:** This is a season of new beginnings—a move to a new place, the birth of a child, a new marriage or relationship, a new job, or simply the joy of a new day. You see great possibilities ahead and want to take full advantage of the best this time has to offer. Because life is looking up, you may want to sprint headlong into your future. But

taking time to be mindful allows you to be intentional about grasping your blessings and good fortune and elevating them even more.

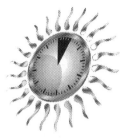 **Day:** You are moving through your happy, routine life. The sun is shining; all is well, maybe even a bit boring. Happiness and even joy may come easily, and people might mistake you for someone who lives a charmed life with no problems. In this season more than any other, you have the capacity to devote emotional energy to introspection because you're not spending it battling difficulties. Meditating during this time will reduce the likelihood of being plunged back into dark and reduce the severity of the impact of the dark season if it arrives.

Be Kind to Yourself

It's okay to jump between the seasons, although you may encounter spoilers in what happens with the four friends illustrating the journey. The primary goal is for you to use the season that meets you where you are at any given moment. And since you can jump around the book, use the graphic images and chapter numbers for each reflection as guideposts for where you are in a particular season.

It's okay if it takes you months or even years to move past a particular reflection. Issues like acknowledging pain, letting go, and forgiveness can take years to address fully. Give yourself permission to go at your own pace.

Don't beat yourself up if your practice ebbs and flows. That's normal. Just keep coming back to it whenever you can.

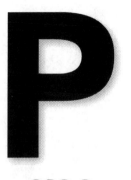

PRACTICE

Reflections to Get You Going

This section provides instructive illustrations to teach you how to practice mindfulness meditation. In this section you will meet Chantelle and Akar, coworkers at Sunderland Medical, Inc. They have a terrible CEO, and their divergent approaches to dealing with their difficult work environment shows you the difference between what might look more like your approach compared to the mindfulness meditation approach.

Chantelle has been meditating for years, and Akar begins because he wants the peace she has. Akar's is not a smooth journey. He doesn't know where to practice, how to sit, or what to think about. Meanwhile, life and work continue to present challenges, and he gets discouraged. Many of us experience Akar's struggles along the path to mindful peace. Be encouraged. Keep learning. Keep moving toward your higher self. Stay on the path!

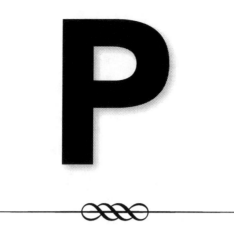

CHAPTER 1
WHY MEDITATION?

"How'd you do it?" Akar Khouri, global vice president of sales, asked the chief legal officer at lunch. They sat under an orange umbrella at a picnic table in a manicured courtyard at Sunderland Medical, Inc. "Gottfried is a lunatic. You're a military wife juggling three kids. How are you so calm?"

Chantelle Dubois smiled sadly. Just then, a man broke from a tour of new employees and hurried over. "Hey, aren't you Vivek Murthy, the former US surgeon general?" he demanded in excitement.

"No!" Akar snapped. "Can't you tell the difference between an Indian and an Egyptian?" The man retreated apologetically.

Chantelle's cheek dimpled. Although Akar was Egyptian and Dr. Murthy was of Indian descent, and their complexions were quite different, Akar did resemble the former surgeon general. His lithe frame, sloped shoulders, regal nose, and distinguished salt-and-pepper hair were strikingly similar. She replied, "I meditate for thirty minutes twice a day."

"And?" Akar asked, raking agitated fingers through his hair.

"That's it. My peace comes from within."

Akar scowled. The French woman continued in her pleasant, accented lilt, "I observe my thoughts and emotions. I choose to hold myself together regardless of events." Chantelle thought about Dale Anderson, her husband, waking up screaming in the middle of the night. She brought herself back to the present.

"I don't have an hour for daily meditation." Akar sighed. "I'm a sales guy. Go, go, go is my mantra."

Five minutes a day can keep the blues at bay. Just start. It adds up.

The Takeaway

Like Akar, many people like the benefits and results of mindfulness meditation but doubt they have time. You invested time in this book, so you obviously care about your wellness. If you don't have time, just start with five minutes each morning. You can do it.

My Journal Reflections

Spend at least five minutes in silent meditation first thing each morning, centering yourself and setting your intentions for the day. Set your alarm for five minutes. You can journal after your five minutes of reflection. It will feel like a long time when you start. But stick with it, and it will get easier.

Day 1.　For the next five minutes, I will imagine how life would be different if I could better weather life's challenges.

Day 2.　Here's how I think mindfulness meditation can help me: _____.

Day 3.　My optimal time of day to practice is _____ because _____.

Day 4.　I can't control people around me, but I can control _____.

Day 5.　Going forward, I will strive to _____.

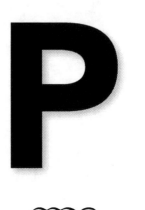

CHAPTER 2

DEBUNKING THE MYTHS

"Isn't mindfulness meditation some weird Eastern mystic crap?" Akar demanded. His deep brown eyes widened in horror as he heard himself voice this long-held bias.

Chantelle's lustrous auburn hair was piled high on her head, and she tucked a stray curl behind her ear as she began. "Many world religions share the same fundamental truths about how to live harmoniously and how to love yourself and others," she said. She explained that while the cultivation of mindfulness stemmed from Buddhist practices, most religions—including Hinduism, Islam, and Christianity—advocated prayer and meditation as core practices.

Akar looked skeptical. "Well, I'm a Christian," he said, looking doubtful.

"Then go find your Bible and count how many times it tells you to meditate."

"So what do I do? Just sit there and empty my mind?" Akar snorted.

"No, that's a myth. You cultivate internal stillness so you can better control and focus your thoughts on positive things."

Akar was still not convinced. "So, if I sit and think positive thoughts, my problems will go away?"

Chantelle's laugh was deep and sonorous. "The world won't stop delivering problems to your doorstep. But you will get much better at handling them from a place of calm, personal power and emotional equilibrium," she explained.

The Takeaway

There are many myths about meditation. It's not a silver bullet or quick fix. But with consistent practice over time, you can reap the benefits.

> Meditation is not about changing others or your environment; it's about transforming your mind and how you see the world.

This journey is not about controlling your terrible boss, that cantankerous spouse, or your badly behaved kids. It's about equipping you with tools and paradigms that will make you better at handling them.

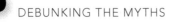

My Journal Reflections

Spend at least five minutes in silent meditation first thing each morning, centering yourself and setting your intentions for the day. Set your alarm for five minutes. You can journal after your five minutes of reflection. It will feel like a long time when you start. But stick with it, and it will get easier.

Day 1.   I will spend five minutes confronting an objection I have to practicing mindfulness meditation. Where did this objection come from, and how can I use this book and the tools I learn to overcome it?

Day 2.   I have long held this negative belief about mindfulness or meditation: _____.

Day 3.   Here are other things I have believed about mindfulness meditation:_____.

Day 4.   Here's what I would like to get from my mindfulness meditation journey: _____.

Day 5.   Here's how I plan to harness the power of mindfulness meditation in my life:_____.

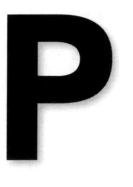

CHAPTER 3

DOES IT REALLY WORK?

"Does this stuff really work, Chantelle?" Akar asked. Today they had lunch by a fountain on Sunderland's campus. The scent of Chantelle's lavender shampoo and the sound of cascading water made Akar feel like he was on vacation.

With a dainty flick of her wrist, Chantelle brushed away sandwich crumbs from the multicolored scarf over her crisp white shirt and then from her navy-blue A-line midi skirt. She told him about Jon Kabat-Zinn, a renowned professor who founded the Stress Reduction Clinic at the University of Massachusetts Medical Center. "His research demonstrated that mindfulness improves both physical and mental health. It helps relieve stress, treat heart disease, improve sleep and self-esteem, and increases one's capacity to deal with difficult life events."

Akar's thick brows rose.

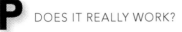

Chantelle continued, "At Harvard Medical School, a neuroscientist and assistant professor of psychology, Dr. Sara Lazar, was the first to document positive changes in brain regions connected to memory, the sense of self, and the regulation of emotions because of mindfulness meditation. Many prestigious universities and Fortune 500 companies, like Apple, Nike, Google, and even the US Army, have incorporated mindfulness meditation into their health and wellness programs.

The Takeaway

Chantelle grazed the tip of the iceberg. There is a growing volume of empirical scientific data demonstrating emotional, physiological, and psychological benefits of mindfulness meditation in people who practice it consistently. Feel free to conduct your own research; talk to those who have practiced it. As one who has pursued the mindfulness meditation path for more than fourteen years at the time of writing this book, I can attest to its effectiveness in alleviating stress and increasing my capacity to better navigate difficult times from a place of calm and personal power. This peace can be yours too. Keep reading.

My Journal Reflections

Spend at least five minutes in silent meditation first thing each morning, centering yourself and setting your intentions for the day. Set your alarm for five minutes. You can journal after your five minutes of reflection. It will feel like a long time when you start. But stick with it, and it will get easier.

Day 1. I will spend the next five minutes just trying to sit in stillness and see how that goes.

Day 2. Based on my research, I have learned this about mindfulness: _____.

Day 3. Based on my research, I have learned this about meditation: _____.

Day 4. Based on what I have learned, I am prepared to take these actions: _____.

Day 5. I will enlist this kind of support to keep my mindfulness meditation practice going: _____.

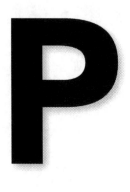

CHAPTER 4

WHEN YOU HAVE NO TIME

"Did you do it?" Chantelle asked Akar the next day.

Akar's dark eyes bounced around the room, and his bronze face blushed. A sheepish look crept across his handsome face. When her wise gaze finally captured his eyes, he couldn't resist blurting out the truth. "I can't take time for mindfulness. My wife insists on a nightly family dinner, the kids get up early, and I must help prepare them for school in the morning."

Chantelle's deep blue eyes twinkled, her sage smile unfaltering. She knew his wife well, Zahra the spitfire.

He threw up his hands. "How can I take time for mindfulness when I never have time for me?"

The Takeaway

Many share Akar's problem. Daily activities crowd our lives, leaving little to no room for self. But taking time for yourself will improve your ability to handle everything else. It also allows you to set your intentions and recenter yourself when unexpected challenges arise.

Give yourself the luxury of time.

Maybe making time means being disciplined enough to wake up at least five minutes earlier every day so you create time to center yourself for the day. Maybe that means taking time before bed or heading for your mindfulness space first thing each morning. It could mean forcing yourself to take a break and not spend your entire lunch hour working at your desk.

Maybe it means going to hide in your mindfulness space for at least five minutes at the end of the day, when the family thinks you are in the bathroom.

Visualize how peaceful you will feel coming out of your mindfulness practice. Visualize how much better and more effective you will be as a friend, employee, spouse, partner, or parent if you give yourself this time. You are worth it.

My Journal Reflections

Spend at least five minutes in silent meditation first thing each morning, centering yourself and setting your intentions for the day. Set your alarm for five minutes. You can journal after your five minutes of reflection.

It will feel like a long time when you start. But stick with it, and it will get easier.

Day 1. I will spend the next five minutes visualizing how I can make space for myself each day this week.

Day 2. I sometimes feel guilty taking time for myself because: _____.

Day 3. The time I have chosen for my 5-minute mindfulness reflection is: _____.

Day 4. I will protect this time and make space for it by: _____.

Day 5. If I miss a day, I will simply endeavor to get back on track because I realize: _____.

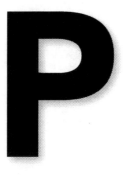

CHAPTER 5

MINDFULNESS MEDITATION DEFINED

Chantelle's slingback kitten heels clipped in short crisp steps as Akar loped along, hands in the pockets of his suit pants. "What is meditation really?"

Chantelle thought a moment. Then she explained, "It is the practice of separating yourself from worldly thoughts and feelings to connect with your inner consciousness."

"And what is mindfulness?" Akar asked.

"Mindfulness is the ability to be fully present in the moment without being overly reactive or overwhelmed by what's happening. You calmly acknowledge your thoughts and feelings without judgment. If you get into the habit of living in the present, you eliminate worrying about the future or trying to revise the past."

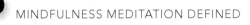

"So should I pretend the past didn't happen and I have no future?" Akar smirked.

Chantelle was patient with her friend, whose slender frame coiled with nervous energy. "No, Akar. Mindfulness is not about ignoring the past or the future. You can acknowledge the past calmly and without judgment and take actions today that will achieve your desired goals for the future. But you can do it without the needless mind-racing anxiety that yields no positive outcomes."

Akar's thick brows threatened to meet above his regal nose. "And you think this stuff really works?"

"Science proves it. Do the research." Chantelle's merry eyes twinkling, she added, "Besides, which of us has been upset by Gottfried the last two days?"

You need not be led around by your and others' emotions.

The Takeaway

Chantelle understands that mindfulness meditation is not about doing but about being, being calm in the presence of upheaval, being confident in who you are as a person born with intention and purpose.

If you are a committed doer like many people and need something to do, create a list of your mindfulness activities each day.

My Journal Reflections

Spend at least five minutes in silent meditation first thing each morning, centering yourself and setting your intentions for the day. Set your alarm for five minutes. You can journal after your five minutes of reflection. It will feel like a long time when you start. But stick with it, and it will get easier.

Day 1.   For the next five minutes, I will examine my emotions about any subject (e.g., work, family, romance) and acknowledge any negative feelings without judgment.

Day 2.   I have negative feelings about: _____.

Day 3.   I am holding on to these negative feelings because: _____.

Day 4.   The reward I get from holding on to my negative feelings is: _____.

Day 5.   Going forward, I will practice letting go of my negative emotions by: _____.

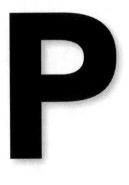

CHAPTER 6

MINDFULNESS VS. MEDITATION

"I'm talking to you. What are you doing?" Chantelle had held up her hand to pause him while she closed her eyes and chewed, and Akar was irritated.

Opening her eyes, she said, "I'm savoring." Akar stared. "I thought you wanted to practice mindfulness. Why aren't you savoring?"

Akar was confused. "I am. I am doing that sitting thing you told me to do daily."

Chantelle laughed. "You are meditating for five minutes each morning, Akar. But you can practice mindfulness all day."

"Well, how about you mindfully mind what I'm saying?" He grumbled.

The Takeaway

To avoid Akar's confusion, it's helpful to understand the difference between mindfulness and meditation. Meditation is what you do to separate yourself from your worldly thoughts and feelings to become fully aware of your inner consciousness. You can use one or more meditative techniques to discipline the mind and increase mental clarity and emotional stability.

Although some use mindfulness as a form of meditation, it doesn't require closed eyes or a quiet space. Its goal is to achieve focused presence in the moment without judgment. It has no religious affiliation. Anyone can do it, no matter what one's beliefs are. Mindfulness can look like:

- Being fully focused on a conversation without your mind wandering, eyes tracking other people going by, or planning what to say next.
- Going within and rebooting even when you are engaged in activity.

Mindful in 5 shows how to combine mindfulness and meditation so you can live and work to your highest and best purpose each day. Begin or end each day by sitting in meditation for five minutes. Then use mindfulness to be fully present in each moment during the remainder of the day.

My Journal Reflections

Spend at least five minutes in silent meditation first thing each morning, centering yourself and setting your intentions for the day. Set your alarm for five minutes. You can journal after your five minutes of reflection.

MINDFULNESS VS. MEDITATION

It will feel like a long time when you start. But stick with it, and it will get easier.

Day 1. I will take the next five minutes to think about how I will use mindfulness meditation to live and work to my highest and best purpose each day.

Day 2. Meditation can help me by: _____.

Day 3. Mindfulness can help me by: _____.

Day 4. I am willing to commit to this practice because:

_____.

Day 5. I hope to gain: _____.

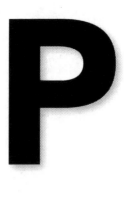

CHAPTER 7

WHERE TO PRACTICE

Akar watched Chantelle in meetings and in interactions with coworkers. He wanted that same peace and focus. As Sunderland Medical's chief legal officer, Chantelle was often Gottfried's target when he raged over the company's performance. Yet, she was unflappable. She sat with her back ramrod straight, sculpted ankles crossed, and chubby fingers gracefully steepled. She spoke her truth gently and with respect, yet with a command that made it clear she knew what she was doing. She even seemed to calm Gottfried. Stepping out of these meetings, her twinkling eyes and winking dimples were contagiously cheerful. Akar wanted that peace and perpetual optimism.

The first night Akar tried meditating, he sat up in bed. But soon he fell asleep. The next morning, he sat on the couch in the living room, but his son and daughter bounded over to play. The next day, he sat on the toilet, but that felt too weird. And his wife, Zahra, fussed at him for hogging the loo. The next day he sat next to the garage door, but something about the feng shui of sitting by the most trafficked door in the house threw off his energy.

"I want a meditation space too," Zahra said. "Why don't we convert the extra bedroom?" The light bulb went on. Ornate Persian tapestries, candles, an altar, cushions, calming pictures. This was the space.

The Takeaway

Like Akar, you may have to try different places to find your ideal meditation spot. It could be a corner, a closet, or an entire room. Create the space that's right for you.

Always return to that space because over time, your body will become conditioned to calm down when you enter your meditation space. As your practice gains momentum, positive vibrations of love and comfort may germinate in your meditation space.

My Journal Reflections

Spend at least five minutes in silent meditation first thing each morning, centering yourself and setting your intentions for the day. Set your alarm for five minutes. You can journal after your five minutes of reflection. It will feel like a long time when you start. But stick with it, and it will get easier.

Day 1.   For the next five minutes, I will find a place in my home that's quiet and that I can return to each day to practice my mindfulness meditation.

Day 2. I picked the "home" spot, where I will return to practice mindfulness meditation when I start my day. Here's where and why: _____.

Day 3. During the day when I'm not home and I need a mindful time-out, here's my plan for where and when I will do it:

_____.

Day 4. I will use these tools to help stay on track (e.g., set a daily alarm/reminder/calendar invite, etc.):

_____.

Day 5. I feel good about my choices and will stick to them by:

_____.

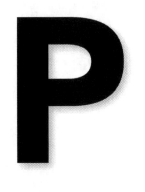

CHAPTER 8
HOW TO MEDITATE

Decorating the room took some negotiations with the ever-opinionated Zahra, but they finally finished. Akar next considered how to get his meditation on. He laid on a cushion but kept falling asleep. He sat cross-legged on the floor, but his flat butt provided no cushion. He tried a lotus pose he often saw on TV, but that was too difficult. Finally, he sat in a chair. Was this an acceptable way to sit?

Five Things

Akar's confusion is understandable since there is no one right way to meditate. But here's a way to start. Start by meditating for five minutes each time. Consistency is more important than length of time. Just get into the habit.

1. Sit in an ergonomically correct posture in the same quiet place each time. You can rest your hands on your thighs and with palms up as a sign of receptivity.

2. Be still. Close your eyes (after you read all the instructions) and relax. Bring your attention to your breath. Don't control your breathing; just mentally watch it go in and out.

3. Use your *Mindful in 5* book to focus your attention on a topic or choose a topic that's germane to your life right now.

4. Vividly visualize the topic and try to keep hold of it. Your thoughts will wander, but this will improve with practice. Never judge or condemn yourself for your wandering mind. Just guide it gently back.

5. When you're done, slowly open your eyes. Immediately notice how you feel. Decide how you want to move through this day or the next.

Repeat the practice daily. Throughout your day, take mindful breaks to take in your surroundings, reflect on how you are feeling, and what's happening in your life without judging it or being overly reactive to it.

My Journal Reflections

Spend at least five minutes in silent meditation first thing each morning, centering yourself and setting your intentions for the day. Set your alarm for five minutes. You can journal after your five minutes of reflection. It will feel like a long time when you start. But stick with it, and it will get easier.

HOW TO MEDITATE

Day 1. For the next five minutes, I will try different positions until I find one I am most comfortable with and that I can assume each time I return to my meditation spot.

Day 2. I decided on this position, described as follows: _____.

Day 3. I chose this position because: _____.

Day 4. Here is my back-up or alternate position when I want a change: _____.

Day 5. I chose this alternative position because: _____.

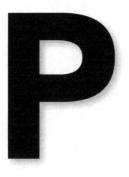

CHAPTER 9

PRACTICE THE SELF-EMBRACE

"The company spent $11 million developing this medical device. We've made promises to investors. The product must launch." The senior marketer, who was chairing the meeting, looked around in defiance.

A junior engineer piped up, "The device has a 25 percent failure rate. We can't kill 25 percent of our customers." Battle lines drawn; a fight erupted among the 18 employees in the meeting. Akar said nothing as the meeting devolved into a shouting match. Finally, he looked across the massive conference room table for Chantelle's reaction.

To his surprise, she was a statue, eyes closed, hands grasping her elbows as if holding herself together. Then she opened her eyes and stood to her full five-foot two inches, piled braided hair adding a foot. Her appearance shimmered in the table's glass surface. She commanded

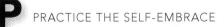

an immediate hush. "Stop talking," she demanded in her strong voice. "First, this conversation goes no further." She looked at the employees with pens poised over notebooks. "Close those," she commanded. Then she began to speak.

In every event and interaction lies a choice, the choice of how we respond. There are always at least two options. The power to choose is yours. And how you use that power defines your growth and freedom.

How to Self-Embrace

Chantelle was practicing the self-embrace. The self-embrace can increase levels of the hormone oxytocin, which can decrease blood pressure, stress, and reduce your heart rate.

When you feel stressed, practice this simple but powerful technique. Close your eyes. Keep your head up or drop it to your chest. Hug yourself and just focus on your breathing. Disconnect from everything to go within and find your peace. You can revisit the day's *Mindful in 5* reflection or decide what to do or say next. You can set a timer, or just do it until you're ready to resume your activities.

My Journal Reflections

Spend at least five minutes in silent meditation first thing each morning, centering yourself and setting your intentions for the day. Set your alarm for five minutes. You can journal after your five minutes of reflection. It will feel like a long time when you start. But stick with it, and it will get easier.

Day 1.   For the next five minutes, I will practice the self-embrace.

Day 2.   My reflections about today's practice:

_____.

Day 3.   What was easy?

_____.

Day 4.   What was challenging?

_____.

Day 5.   Here's how I will incorporate the self-embrace into my day: _____.

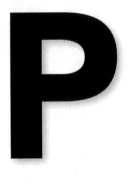

CHAPTER 10

PRACTICE
NONJUDGMENT

"Can you believe our sales system crashed? This is awful!" Akar said, smearing beads of sweat across his brow.

"Is it?" Chantelle asked. Akar glared. "Consider practicing nonjudgment," Chantelle suggested, nonplussed.

"What?" Akar asked, annoyed.

Chantelle told him this tale:

> A farmer with a large tract only had an old mule to plough it. "How sad," his neighbors clucked.
>
> The farmer said, "In all things, I am grateful."

Then one day the mule died. "How awful," his neighbors cried.

"Is it?" the farmer asked.

While walking his tract, the farmer discovered a badly beaten man under a hedge. "This is awful," cried his neighbors. "Leave him lest the bandits return!"

"Is it awful?" the farmer asked while nursing the man to health. It turned out the man was wealthy, and he sent the farmer a young stallion in thanks.

"Fantastic," yelled the fickle neighbors. "Good thing you helped him!"

"Was it?" asked the farmer."

When the farmer's son visited, he was riding the steed when it was spooked and bucked. The son fell on his head and died instantly.

"Oh no," cried the neighbors. "This is the worst!"

"Is it?" the farmer asked. "In all things, I am grateful." His daughter-in-law told him his son had a disease and was dying a slow, painful death. His son's worst fear had been the horrifying path that lay ahead.

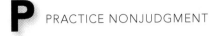

The Takeaway

Many of us are like the farmer's neighbors and rush to label situations. A core tenet of mindfulness is nonjudgment.

Acceptance without judgment recognizes that things just are. Each event wasn't inherently good or bad. It just was.

Being present without judgment includes resisting the urge to label events because all things work together in complex patterns that are difficult—if not impossible—to define in a single dimension.

My Journal Reflections

Spend at least five minutes in silent meditation first thing each morning, centering yourself and setting your intentions for the day. Set your alarm for five minutes. You can journal after your five minutes of reflection. It will feel like a long time when you start. But stick with it, and it will get easier.

Day 1.   For the next five minutes, I will think of a time when I thought something good or bad happened that turned out not to be.

Day 2.   I thought a wonderful thing happened that turned out not to be when: _____.

Day 3. I thought a bad thing happened that turned out not to be when: _____.

Day 4. Right now, I have placed a value judgement on: _____.

Day 5. Going forward, I will take each day as it comes and resist defining events by: _____.

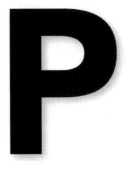

CHAPTER 11

THE POWER OF MANTRAS

Every morning after brushing her teeth, Chantelle settles herself cross-legged on the meditation pillow in their glass sunroom. Today she rubs her bruised shin, where Dale kicked her during a nightmare. The first big challenge after they married was meshing her French and his American cultures. Dale suffers from post-traumatic stress disorder. Behind the façade of the happy military couple with three adorable boys and lovely suburban home lies pain. Chantelle adores Dale; he is the bravest man she knows. He has weathered the worst of heavy combat. She respects his dedication to country, but the cost to him and their family is dear.

With palms on her thighs, she closes her eyes and mentally watches her breath. She inhales peace and exhales stress. She repeats a short phrase in her mind: "I choose love. I choose joy and peace this day."

With each repetition she focuses on the deeper meaning of each word. She visualizes herself treating Dale with love and compassion. She sees herself facing her volatile CEO, Gottfried, with calm. Sometimes it takes a long time to clearly visualize her intentions.

The Takeaway

Chantelle uses the power of intention to influence her daily actions. You can too.

First we think, then we do, then we become.

Mindfulness meditation is less about doing and mostly about becoming—becoming calm and empowered from within no matter what's happening out there. It is about coming into the fullness of all the gifts you were born with.

The trouble for many of us is that we have been tricked into believing we are less than we are through repetitive negative messaging. Harness the same power of repetitive messaging to transform negative into positive belief systems.

My Journal Reflections

Spend at least five minutes in silent meditation first thing each morning, centering yourself and setting your intentions for the day. Set your alarm for five minutes. You can journal after your five minutes of reflection.

It will feel like a long time when you start. But stick with it, and it will get easier.

Day 1.   I will take the next five minutes to choose a mantra and repeat it, going deeper into its meaning with every repetition.

Day 2.   Today I am going to choose this mantra because: _____.

Day 3.   Until now I have been repeating the following negative statements in my head: _____.

Day 4.   Regardless of where the negative statements came from, I relinquished them today because I recognize: _____.

Day 5.   Going forward, I will replace my negative thought habits with positive ones by: _____.

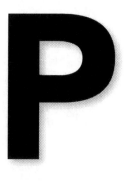

CHAPTER 12

FIVE MINUTES IS FOREVER

Akar dragged himself into the meditation room. He was drained. His pants sagged over his flat bottom, his tie was crooked, and even his thick salt-and pepper silver hair fell limp. But when he entered the room, he instantly felt a sense of calm positive energy. He had meditated in the morning but was glad he returned that night.

He read a bit and then set his alarm for five minutes. He began with deep-breathing exercises, inhaling, holding the breath, exhaling.

After three or four repetitions, he was ready for his reflection. To counteract Gottfried's negativity, he chose a chant. With each repetition, he dug deeper and visualized how he would move through the day from a place of self-trust.

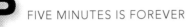

It started out well enough but quickly derailed. *I trust my judgment. I trust my judgment. Chantelle is out of town. I'll eat lunch at my desk. No, I should take a mindful break.* Then he caught himself. *Oh, wait, I trust my judgment. I trust my judgment. I'll stop by the grocery store, so I can take sandwiches to work. Oh wait, I trust my judgment.*

After forever, he thought, *my alarm is broken because I've been struggling for an hour!* He waited for the alarm to sound. Finally, Akar peeked and realized it had only been two minutes!

The Takeaway

Akar's is a common experience. Five minutes feels like forever, and it's a fight to discipline your thoughts. Don't be discouraged. Even seasoned meditators have days like this. With time and consistency, it gets easier. If you spend the entire time fighting distraction, simply think, *Self, I didn't do so well today, but I'll be back to try again.* Master the art of showing up consistently, and the rest will take care of itself.

My Journal Reflections

Spend at least five minutes in silent meditation first thing each morning, centering yourself and setting your intentions for the day. Set your alarm for five minutes. You can journal after your five minutes of reflection. It will feel like a long time when you start. But stick with it, and it will get easier.

Day 1. For the next five minutes, I will visualize myself overcoming every obstacle to return to my meditation space every morning at the same time.

Day 2.   I will practice mindfulness meditation at this time every day: _____.

Day 3.   I will practice mindfulness meditation in this location every day:_____.

Day 4.   Here are the distractions I think will be most challenging for me to overcome: _____.

Day 5.   Here are the steps I will take to minimize the impact of those distractions so I can continue my mindfulness meditation practice: _____.

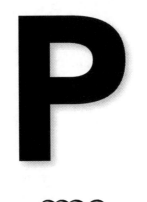

THE BENEFITS OF MEDITATION

"Chantelle, this meditation thing is hard," Akar said, happy his friend was back as he loped beside her. He was suited up for a client meeting and tried meditation beforehand. But he kept worrying about the meeting.

"The hardest part is establishing the habit and sticking to it," Chantelle said.

Flashes of Chantelle's composure in myriad difficult situations flew through Akar's mind. With a new openness he said, "Remind me why I'm doing this again."

Chantelle rearranged her bright scarf against her black dress. She didn't miss a beat. "Cambridge University studied the benefits of mindfulness meditation and found that it can reduce the symptoms of subclinical depression and anxiety. And it can substantially reduce stress.

The Mayo Clinic found that meditation can reduce stress and negative emotions, increase focus, awareness, patience, and tolerance." Lots of supporting science and lots of room to benefit you."

The Takeaway

Benefits vary and depend on consistent practice. Studies have shown that you can reap great benefits of meditation with as few as twelve minutes a day and ideally, twenty to thirty minutes once or twice a day over an extended period. Meditation is not a quick fix; it is a daily journey of becoming. The benefits cited by scientists and proponents of the practice are real and can be yours with consistency and practice.

Don't be discouraged if it doesn't feel like anything is happening. Grass grows even though you can't see the process. Just start with five minutes each morning. Some days will feel like you're fighting to be still every second. Other days you will feel the warm bliss of meditation and won't want to stop. Let the blissful days fuel the hard days. And above all else, just keep at it.

My Journal Reflections

Spend at least five minutes in silent meditation first thing each morning, centering yourself and setting your intentions for the day. Set your alarm for five minutes. You can journal after your five minutes of reflection. It will feel like a long time when you start. But stick with it, and it will get easier.

Day 1.   For the next five minutes, I will reflect on what I hope to gain from mindfulness meditation.

Day 2. Through my practice, I hope to become:

_____.

Day 3. Because mindfulness meditation is a journey not a destination, I will maintain consistency by:

_____.

Day 4. Even when I am discouraged, I will keep going because: _____.

Day 5. To resist the temptation to watch the grass grow, I will focus on: _____.

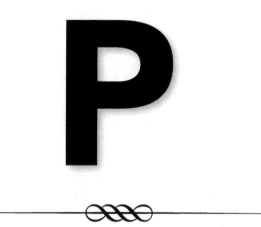

CHAPTER 14
NOTHING IS HAPPENING

"Why do you look like someone stole your dance moves and hit the stage first?" Chantelle asked Akar.

"Nothing's happening," Akar lamented. "I've been at this meditation thing for three months, and nothing's changed. I love them to bits, but Zahra and the kids still get on my nerves, and Gottfried's still tirading. I wanted to feel unflappable like you, but it's not happening." He sat down heavily on the bright blue bench near the Sunderland campus auditorium and rolled up his shirt sleeves. Slouching in discouragement, he said, "Maybe this meditation thing just isn't for me."

Chantelle patted his forearm. "You're doing great, Akar. You just can't see it," she said. When he looked at her skeptically, Chantelle asked, "When was the last time you felt really upset about Gottfried?"

Akar paused. It had been weeks.

The Takeaway

The internal evolution of becoming isn't obvious to the becomer. Akar didn't realize it, but over time, he was less upset every time Gottfried threw a tantrum. Gottfried hadn't changed, but Akar's reaction did. Akar also didn't notice that even when he did get upset, the peaks of his anxiety were less pronounced. Only when Chantelle pointed it out did Akar see the change.

Practicing mindfulness is like physical exercise. You don't see your muscles develop, but one day you flex, and there they are. Also, the more you practice, the stronger your concentration and focus become, and the less you are buffeted by the daily ups and downs of life. Don't stare at your mental biceps each day, looking for signs of growth. Just focus on the discipline of showing up every day and taking time for yourself. The results will come in time. Five minutes gets you started. The greater your consistency and concentration, the better your results.

My Journal Reflections

Spend at least five minutes in silent meditation first thing each morning, centering yourself and setting your intentions for the day. Set your alarm for five minutes. You can journal after your five minutes of reflection. It will feel like a long time when you start. But stick with it, and it will get easier.

Day 1.   I will spend the next five minutes taking stock of how long I have been practicing mindfulness meditation and how consistent my efforts have been.

Day 2. I will focus on showing up during the following days and times this month for my mindfulness meditation practice: _____.

Day 3. Next week I will commit the following days and times to my mindfulness meditation practice: _____.

Day 4. Here are the benefits I hope to gain from my mindfulness meditation practice: _____.

Day 5. I will avoid obsessing over my progress by simply focusing on: _____.

THE

SEASONS

OF

YOUR

LIFE

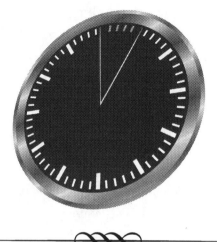

DARK

Finding the Light When Darkness Has Fallen

The meditations in this season are best used when you are experiencing difficulties in life. You were afraid a storm was gathering on the horizon, but you were wrong; it was a full-blown hurricane! In the dark of your life's night, those things that were sliding sideways plunged into what felt like your own valley of the shadow of death:

- A global pandemic derailed your life.
- That bad relationship progressed into an ugly and permanent breakup.
- The financial clouds rolling in over the horizon have blown up into gales of financial destruction.
- You finally went to the doctor, and the diagnosis was worse than everything you feared.
- You lost your job or a loved one passed away.

Join our mindfulness support group in which four strangers become friends. Each has a personal struggle that drove them to join the group.

- Barry is struggling to accept the demise of his marriage.
- Singita is trying to cope with difficult family relationships.
- Rashad and Brianna celebrated their twins heading off to college. Now what?

Hopefully you will see your struggles in the journeys of the four and how you can harness the power of mindfulness meditation to face the ups and downs of each day.

The Dark season is when many people are most vulnerable and most likely to retreat into a shell, forsaking daily routines and good habits. And this is the time when it is most beneficial to spend energy on mindfulness meditation.

Take comfort in knowing that you're not the first person to encounter difficulty or to struggle. Like these four friends, hopefully you will come to see that it's not what's happening out there that defines you. It is what's between your own two ears.

Use the reflections in this dark season to help you step into your new paradigm of self-empowerment and hope, no matter what is happening in your life.

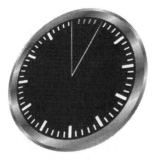

CHAPTER 1

TAKE TIME

Barry Miles instinctively grabbed for his five-year-old son as the plane instantly dropped ten feet. "Weeee!" squealed little Navesh in delight. After another ten feet, passengers began screaming and crying. A storm pummeled the plane, tossing the jetliner about like a sparrow.

The captain's reassuring voice beamed through the intercom. "We are experiencing significant turbulence and loss of cabin pressure. Oxygen masks above your seat will deploy. Please place the mask on first, and then assist other passengers."

Barry looked at his son. The gleeful child turned wailing boy mirrored the palpable terror of the fellow passengers. Navesh began hyperventilating and wheezing, his asthma kicking in.

Ignoring his own mask and the dizziness on the edges of his consciousness, Barry reached for his son. He didn't appreciate how fast

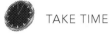

the air was changing in the cabin and that he only had seconds to put his mask on to feed oxygen to his brain. Just as he pulled down his son's mask, hypoxia overcame him, and everything faded to black.

The Takeaway

> If you are not good to yourself, you may be no good to others.

Barry's experience is not uncommon, especially for parents. Many people view time as a luxury. Taking time for yourself is not selfish, and you should not feel guilty about it. It is especially important in your darkest season, when you need to be most centered to weather storms that could destabilize you. Ensuring your own wellness is also the best assurance that you will be able to serve others.

In this moment, be present with yourself. Each of us receives the same twenty-four hours each day. If you spend eight to twelve hours working, isn't it only fair that you take at least five minutes for yourself? Be still. For yourself. Right now.

My Journal Reflections

Spend at least five minutes in silent meditation first thing each morning for at least five days this week. Be intentional in committing to your meditation habit in this sunny season.

Day 1. For the next five minutes, I will give myself the gift of time to just be still and breathe.

Day 2. I feel pressured to give all my time away by:

_____.

Day 3. I give myself an average of this much time daily because: _____.

Day 4. Ideally, I want to give myself this much time daily: _____.

Day 5. Here is my plan for creating and protecting the space for my personal care time: _____.

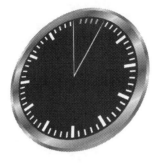

CHAPTER 2
SHOW UP

Cassie watched Singita, the beautiful, petite Indian woman, manipulate a completely jumbled Rubik's Cube with speed that blurred her long red fingernails and the multicolored squares. Singita had arrived early. Cassie was leader of the Mindful in 5 peer support group, which provided a haven to work through difficult transitions. Today was their first meeting.

Cassie was a tall, pale ruler of a woman whose vaguely ginger curls contrasted to the fiery red buzz cut Barry Miles wore when he burst into the room. A taut barrel on broomsticks, Barry was broad and chiseled. His every movement declared prior military training, now a little soft. "Hi, y'all," he said as he flashed open his coat to blind everyone with an enormous belt buckle declaring "Texas." Red plaid shirt, faded jeans, and large furry boots completed the ensemble.

Cassie pretended not to notice as he appraised her flowy flannel shirt and skirt. It was dusty brown today, but she had the same outfit in camouflage green and slate gray. Only her intelligent green eyes with flecks of shooting amber and her conflagration of curls that she tried to tame in a knot at the nape of her neck gave away the fire within her.

After Barry came Nandi Chaya, Fiona Darby, and Jillian and Gene Adams. Their gait and clothing created impressions before they ever spoke.

The Takeaway

You may have heard the adage, "You never get a second chance to make a first impression." As the group session opens, we see how different individuals show up in the same room.

And so it is the same with each of us. The impressions we make are defined by how we show up in the world. Even as Cassie watched her new group members show up, she was making her own impressions on them and they on her.

My Journal Reflections

Spend at least five minutes in silent meditation first thing each morning for at least five days this week. Mindfulness is about being present in the moment without judgment. If on reflection you don't like certain aspects of how you show up, develop a plan to make positive changes.

Day 1.   For the next five minutes, I will consider how often I am timely when I show up for events at work or in my personal life.

Day 2.   When I show up at work, I want to convey the following: _____.

Day 3.   When I show up with my family, I want to convey the following: _____.

Day 4.   When I show up with my friends, I want to convey the following: _____.

Day 5.   Based on the feedback I have received; I'd like to change this one thing about how I show up in the world: _____.

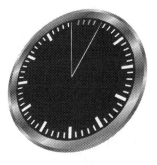

CHAPTER 3

THWARTED EXPECTATIONS

At six o'clock, Cassie cleared her throat and welcomed the eight seated attendees. As she spoke, the last four stragglers scuttled in and quickly took their seats. She pushed her large tortoiseshell glasses up her nose and announced in her smooth voice, "We'll begin with five minutes of silent meditation. Sit in an ergonomically correct posture, torso upright, feet planted firmly on the floor." Cassie glanced around the circle to check her students' postures. Everyone's feet were planted firmly on the floor except for Singita's, which swung merrily to and fro. Singita sat with eyes closed, oblivious to her own movement. The now perfectly solved Rubik's Cube rested in her lap, blending into her salwar kameez, a splash of fresh color in the pale room.

After meditation, Singita volunteered to go first. "Hi, my name is Singita Patel." Cassie's curls bobbed, accompanied by an encouraging smile.

"Hi, Singita," everyone said in unison.

Singita shifted, looking uncomfortable. "I-I …" She tried again. "I lost my appä, my father."

Cassie looked sympathetic. "I am so sorry. Recently?"

Singita's large black eyes grew. She shook her head, rich dark ponytail bouncing as if trying to escape. "No. Well, he's not dead, but I lost him." Her eyes downcast, Singita muttered, "He always treated me badly. I didn't deserve it. I shouldn't be going through this!"

The group listened. Some looked on quizzically and others sympathetically.

The Takeaway

Like Singita, many of us have thwarted expectations. Our parents fall short, our jobs are not fulfilling, and our lives aren't what we wanted. How can we minimize this suffering? First, check your expectations. Thwarted expectations are often the root of disappointment. Accept what you can't control; you especially can't control other people. And be introspective. Understand your own motivations that fuel unmet expectations and disappointments.

My Journal Reflections

Spend at least five minutes in silent meditation first thing each morning for at least five days this week. Use these topics and your journal to guide your thoughts about the quality of your relationships this week.

Day 1.   For the next five minutes I will consider a relationship or situation I am disappointed in.

Day 2.   I am harboring these unmet expectations about my situation: _____.

Day 3.   I believe I should be exempt from this suffering because: _____.

Day 4.   Since I am unhappy, I would prefer that things were different in this way: _____.

Day 5.   I can avoid this pain in future in a constructive and positive way by: _____.

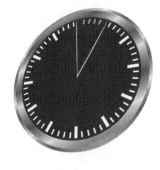

CHAPTER 4

ESCAPING PAIN

Singita seemed still, but her ponytail trembled. "I think Appä always believed his friends and neighbors were beneath him. After I obeyed his command to apply for his US citizenship, he denounced everyone in our small community in Chennai. When the immigration application was denied, he disowned me, forcing Ammä, my brother, and sisters to choose sides."

Unable to continue, Singita lapsed into silence. Her perfectly sculpted brows flattened into a scowl that contorted her smooth, honey-hued face. The group sat in stunned silence while Cassie made sure Singita had no more to say.

Then she began. "In the Disney movie *Finding Nemo,* there is a scene where the father, Marlon, is searching for his son, Nemo. A school of fish tell his sidekick, Dory, that when they arrive at this trench, they should swim through it, not over it."

Cassie noted Singita's confusion and continued. "The trench is deep and scary-looking, complete with skeletons of long-dead fish. Marlon takes one look and decides they should swim over it. Over Dory's objections, he tricks her into going over it to the bright, sun-drenched sea overhead. The flaw in Marlon's escapism is almost immediately apparent, when the two little fish are beset by a swarm of venomous jellyfish."

Surviving a breakup or dealing with an involuntary life change is a lot like this. There you sit, facing a menacing trench of agony, disgruntlement, embarrassment, disillusionment, and a ball in your stomach of negative feelings you can't even put into words.

Like Singita, you have a choice. Do you evade the trench? Surely the blue skies of alcohol, new relationships, retail therapy, or even drug addiction are easier than going through that trench. Right?

My Journal Reflections

Spend at least five minutes in silent meditation first thing each morning for at least five days this week. Clarifying your true desire may be harder than you think.

Day 1.   For the next five minutes I will stare down that terror, rage, disappointment, blame, self-doubt, and all the emotions I have been experiencing. And breathe.

Day 2.   This   is   what   my   trench   looks like: _____.

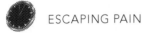

Day 3. Here's how I feel about my trench:

    _____.

Day 4. I am most frightened of going through the trench because: _____.

Day 5. The negative consequences of my going over the trench are: _____.

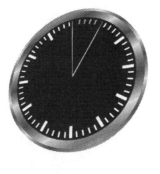

CHAPTER 5

FACE PAIN

"What's wrong with pain avoidance?" Barry demanded. "Between car racin', rodeo, and, and," Barry caught himself as he saw the women glaring, "well, you can drown a lot of pain!" Beside him, Rashad Patterson guffawed while his wife, Brianna, glowered.

"Barry, right?" Cassie asked.

"Yup. Barry Andrew Miles. *Bam!* From Danville, Kentucky."

Singita frowned. "Your belt screams Texas."

"I wish I was from Texas!" Barry slapped a big hairy hand on his big solid thigh, and gales of laughter shook his robust frame.

Cassie continued, "It might seem easier. But soon the venomous jellyfish of negative consequences from addictions, avoidance, and your own unresolved negative emotions sting. Emotional recovery varies for everyone. And there's no shortcut."

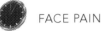

Cassie surveyed the group. Tugging her shapeless shirt, she said, "Years ago, I got divorced." There were surprised gasps from the attendees.

Cassie nodded. "Shocking! I'm such a nice person, how could that possibly happen? I get that all the time. It's why I became a counselor. My DivorceCare coach said it could take half the length of the relationship to get over it. I was married for fifteen years. What?" Cassie smiled at the slack jaws.

"I was single for ten years before I remarried. Determined never to encounter the divorce trench again, I took the time to heal and become this woman, to shed my negative cycles, and attract the kind of relationship I wanted. My goal is to turn all of you into mindful ninjas so you can each conquer your trench. Going through that scary trench for all those years paid off in more ways than I could have ever dreamed."

The Takeaway

You attract what you reflect.

Cassie is happily married to her soul mate, Alan. What she gained from going through the trench was priceless. Don't go over the trench. Go through it.

My Journal Reflections

Spend at least five minutes in silent meditation first thing each morning for at least five days this week. Decide this week that no matter how difficult, you will face your journey through pain head-on.

Day 1.   For the next five minutes, I will devise a plan for going through my pain.

Day 2.   This happened in my life to bring me to this situation: _____.

Day 3.   I want my life to change for the better in these ways: _____.

Day 4.   Here are the trusted and willing people I can lean on while I go through my pain: _____.

Day 5.   Realistically, it may take this long to get through my pain: _____.

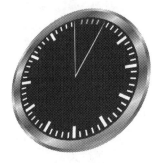

CHAPTER 6
COPING

Brianna yelped in surprise as fur slithered around her dainty ankles. Shadow The Cat hissed as Cassie scooped him up. With a bite-sized chunk missing from one ear, pink crepe skin exposed by patches of missing gray fur, the cat looked as if he'd lost a battle with one of his bigger cousins. With his one insolent eye, the cat blinked at Brianna. Brianna shuddered. "You call that thing Shadow?" she asked.

"Shadow The Cat," said Cassie.

"Shadow?"

"Shadow The Cat," said Cassie.

Brianna let it go. "That's why we're here. We need a way through the trench." Her smile was brittle from years of bristling at her husband. "Our twins left for college. The transition is … difficult."

Rashad chimed in, "Yeah, eighteen years ago Brianna went from being a wife to a mom, and that's all she's been since." His grin belied the bite in his tone. "Now that she's lost the kids, she wants her husband back." His amber eyes blazed as he patted her limp hand resting in his with angry vigor. Cassie quirked a brow.

"Funny," said Barry, cocking his head, "you look like the perfect Black suburban couple. I'd have never guessed y'all got marital problems."

The Takeaway

How do you maintain calm in the face of negative changes you can't control?

Control what you can and let go of the rest.

Accept what you can't control. Brianna and Rashad couldn't prevent their twins from growing up. Identify small and big things you can do in response to any given situation and do them. Brianna and Rashad can rediscover each other and their marriage—if they both want to.

Once you identify what you can do, put a plan in place for accomplishing your aspirations. Once you have a plan, stop worrying about events you can't control.

My Journal Reflections

Spend at least five minutes in silent meditation first thing each morning for at least five days this week. It's easy to read this week's reflections, but some of them may be difficult to get your head around. Return to them as often as necessary and lean into your journaling to help you.

Day 1.   For the next five minutes I will scroll through events that have worried me without judgment and consider how they made me feel.

Day 2.   Here is the one thing I'm most worried about right now: _____.

Day 3.   Here's what I'd like to see happen to address it: _____.

Day 4.   Here's what (if anything) I can do to help: _____.

Day 5.   Here's how I'm going to let go of what I can't control: _____,

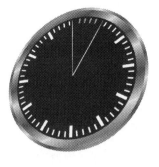

CHAPTER 7

FINANCIAL WORRIES

Barry's broad chest constricted as he stared at the child support calculation for his sons. They were only seven and five years old; he'd go bankrupt! He felt so positive when he left the last group session that he thought nothing could touch him. But now he yearned for a drink, even after a decade of sobriety.

He could scarcely afford the divorce lawyer who sent him this proposal, and these numbers represented the best-case scenario. Ironically, as a lawyer himself, he understood how costly a support battle would be. His father-in-law, Mr. Gupta, was wealthy, Indian, and had never liked him. His eldest daughter marrying a Caucasian was a deep insult. Burying Barry in a mountain of expenses would delight him. Barry would have difficulty paying his bills, and that was before his three useless brothers called to mooch, which they always did. Barry placed the document facedown and walked away. *I can't think about this right now,* he decided.

The Takeaway

Finances can be stressful. Fights about money are still touted as a key contributor to divorce. Sometimes life takes an unexpected turn. A divorce, job loss, pandemic, medical diagnosis, an accident, or a death in the family can move you from financial stability to insecurity overnight.

Being mindful about money management includes understanding your motivations and being intentional about your spending. This is especially true when faced with a significant financial hurdle.

You can't address what you don't face.

First, face the problem head-on and quantify it. There are many books, guides, and tools that cover every aspect of financial planning. Whether you are digging yourself out of a hole or coasting to financial independence, there are resources to assist you. Take the first mindful step to move from fear to fiscal peace today.

My Journal Reflections

Spend at least five minutes in silent meditation first thing each morning for at least five days this week. No matter your financial situation, there is something you can do this week to improve it.

Day 1. I will take the next five minutes to contemplate my current financial situation, what's working and what's not. I will do this without judgment or angst.

Day 2. I resent being placed in financial difficulty because:
_____.

Day 3. I recognize I am where I am financially because:
_____.

Day 4. I will take these steps to address my biggest financial challenge: _____.

Day 5. I will take these steps to foster financial contentment with my situation: _____.

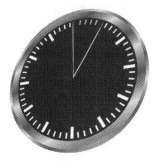

CHAPTER 8

HARBORING RESENTMENT

Six days after their last group-counseling session and one day before their next session, Brianna was still angry. For the entire week the only words spoken between her and her husband, Rashad, were necessary administrative comments like, "Did you remember to pick up the dry cleaning?"

As she braided her beautiful mane into cornrows for the night, Brianna tried to be present, but her mind kept returning to Rashad. She didn't want to go to the session. She felt so embarrassed and humiliated by what Rashad had said. He made it sound like for eighteen years, she had done nothing for him; she had been just a mother monster. How dare he!

The Takeaway

Sometimes we are so affronted by the words and actions of others that we can't see past it. This is especially true when those people are close to us, such as family members, coworkers, and friends.

During her morning meditations (yes, it took many sessions), Brianna came to accept a few realities. As much as she would like to, she couldn't control her husband's perspective on their marriage. She could only change her reactions, attitudes, and how she treated Rashad.

Brianna also reflected on her own behavior, the years she forgot their anniversary, the times she was too tired for intimacy after long days driving the kids around (even though Rashad was there too), how she snapped at him when she was tired (which was often), and how every sarcastic, denigrating comment she had made now stood between them like a moat of spikes, and she couldn't get through. No wonder he was filled with resentment!

Done with her hair, her long fingers drummed the dresser. She could see the negative patterns but wondered if they could be fixed.

My Journal Reflections

Spend at least five minutes in silent meditation first thing each morning for at least five days this week. Use these topics and your journal to guide your thoughts.

Day 1. I am harboring resentment over: _____.

Day 2. My intention in holding on to my bitterness is to punish: _____.

Day 3.   I can see that my resentment is costing me:

_____.

Day 4.   If I continue along this path, I can foresee the following
outcomes: _____.

Day 5.   Starting today, I will begin to change:

_____.

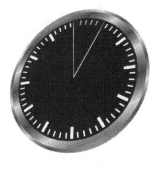

CHAPTER 9
REJECT SELF-DOUBT

As she did every Sunday evening, Singita faced her siblings on her computer screen. In birth order, Sarani, Salma, Sameena, and Bhakti, the youngest, looked back. The middle child, Singita, pulled her sisters together weekly.

"I don't understand why Appä disowned me. What was so wrong with me?" Singita asked.

"You mean why not Bhakti the tramp?" asked Sarani smacking on her mango, juice dribbling down her chubby chin.

"Hey!" Bhakti's black eyes blazed.

"Well, you did refuse to send him money and move to California to marry that wealthy Indian fellow. Screwing up Appä's immigration application was the last straw," Sarani said, nonplussed. "You weren't a very good girl now, were you? And there you sit, alone, unmarried, and unloved."

Singita's eyes burned with old fury. "I didn't refuse," she shot back, "I didn't have the money! And that guy was a waiter living in a slum. I didn't screw up Appä's immigration application. I even hired a lawyer, but it was denied!" She raged on. But secretly, Singita wondered about the truth in Sarani's biting remarks.

The Takeaway

Sometimes negative self-talk is so baked into our internal dialogues and enforced by those closest to us that we don't even notice it. Then over time, it becomes part of the normal wallpaper lining the halls of our minds, and we walk past it daily without even noticing how garish and ugly it is. And much of this negative self-talk is untrue.

We too readily accept the negative lies
embedded in our minds about ourselves.

Without blame, identify negative thought habits that have embedded themselves in your psyche. We often become what we think. Calling yourself unworthy, old, stupid, and so on, or accepting these labels from others, may become your reality.

Decide today not to give more space to the ugly thoughts.

My Journal Reflections

Spend at least five minutes in silent meditation first thing each morning for at least five days this week. Don't accept the first or even the second answer your brain throws at you for the lies you have accepted. Dig deep; there's more lurking back there. Start with five minutes, but ruminate on this one, and more will come to you.

Day 1.   I will take the next five minutes to identify the biggest lie I have accepted about myself.

Day 2.   Here is how it manifests in my life:

_____.

Day 3.   It has prevented me from:

_____.

Day 4.   I reject the lie because I know that:

_____.

Day 5.   Whenever that lie resurfaces, I will redirect my thoughts by:

_____.

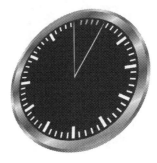

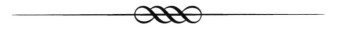

CHAPTER 10
CONFRONT ANXIETY

Brianna lay awake worrying about many things. Who was she without her children? Was Rashad right when he said all she had been the past eighteen years was a mother? Did she really treat her husband more like a utility player than a partner? Did she even want a partner? The last question snuck up on her, making her shudder as she mentally batted it away.

It was 2 o'clock in the morning, and Brianna and Rashad's children had only been gone a month. She was happy they were thriving and finding their way at college, and she couldn't do anything about their departure. But she could do something about her relationship with Rashad. She rolled over to face him as he lay snoring gently.

She used to love watching him sleep. But now, not even his distinguished gray temples or smooth caramel pores caught her attention.

"Rashad, Rashad." He grunted and shifted. She put a hand on his arm. "Can we talk?" Rashad opened a single bleary eye and regarded her warily.

The Takeaway

Many of us are like Brianna. We lay awake at night, worries racing through our minds that balloon into giant fears with no solution. We worry about our jobs, our children, our relationships, the things we wish hadn't happened, and the things we are afraid will happen. Worries are like indecisive squirrels in the face of oncoming traffic. They run hither and yon with no direction and lead to no resolution.

Research shows that excessive worrying can have a negative impact on your relationships, sleep, job performance, and health.

One question to confront your anxiety is whether you can fix the subject of your worries right now. Do you have control over what's worrying you? If so, can you address it right this minute?

My Journal Reflections

Spend at least five minutes in silent meditation first thing each morning for at least five days this week. Don't worry about the fact that you have worries. Breathe through them.

Day 1.   For the next five minutes I will mentally confront the top three things I am most worried about. I will not judge myself for worrying about them but just acknowledge my concerns.

Day 2. Of the things I thought of yesterday, I am most worried about: _____.

Day 3. Of the one thing I am most worried about, here are aspects of it that I can control: _____.

Day 4. Of the one thing I am most worried about, here are aspects of it I cannot control: _____.

Day 5. I will take these three steps to address the source of my anxiety: _____.

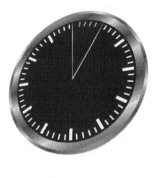

CHAPTER 11

REPLACE ANXIETY

"I feel like we've drifted apart," Brianna began. Her husband said nothing. "I'd like to return to how things were when we started dating."

Rashad propped himself up on one elbow. "Oh, you mean back to the wonderful days when you got everything you wanted? When I ran behind you, always chasing and never satisfied? Back when I needed you more than you ever wanted me?" Brianna was taken aback. Rashad opened the floodgates. He was a brilliant engineer and had evidently catalogued everything he had ever been unhappy about in their marriage.

This wasn't how she envisioned this conversation going at all! There she was, trying to address a worry she could do something about like their support group leader, Cassie, taught them. But rather than alleviating her anxiety, her effort to confront the problem exacerbated it, adding a new beehive of stinging worries over the survival of her marriage.

The Takeaway

Life is imperfect. Sometimes the actions we take to address a problem seem to make it worse. It doesn't mean the original intent was wrong. But as in Brianna's case, people and situations can react in unexpected ways.

Rather than allowing unexpected twists to add to your anxiety, you can still replace the worry habit. Habits of thought are more powerful than habits of behavior because:

First we think, then we do, then we become.

Changing thought habits is incredibly difficult in part because thoughts travel down well-defined neural pathways that grow stronger with repetition, just like your physical muscles grow stronger with exercise. So rather than gritting your teeth and trying to muscle your way out of a negative thought habit, it may be easier to simply focus on replacing the worry thought habit with a new habit.

My Journal Reflections

Spend at least five minutes in silent meditation first thing each morning for at least five days this week. Get serious about defeating your negative thought habits no matter how long it takes and however many times you need to return to these reflections.

Day 1. For the next five minutes, I will think of something that worries me and practice replacing the worrisome thought with a positive one.

Day 2. Every time I start worrying about it, I will replace it with: _____.

Day 3. I could carry around a notepad and write down each worry to make it more tangible and, therefore, smaller so I can address it. I will do this because_____, or use this other method to tame worrisome thoughts: _____.

Day 4. Here are the aspects of my worrisome issue I can control: _____.

Day 5. I will address this concern by: _____.

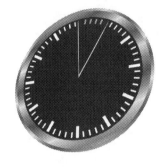

CHAPTER 12

PRACTICE SELF-LOVE

Singita was frustrated. All day a single thought had been tormenting her, *I am not enough. Appä knows it, and my sisters do too.* Over multiple meditative reflections, she realized she had been carrying this lie since childhood. It was so embedded in her psyche that she never questioned or even recognized it was there. It took a lot of introspection and going step-by-step through her personal history to identify times when that thought rooted itself more deeply or when it influenced her outward behavior.

The origin of this lie didn't reside in any single event but in statements and insinuations from family members that were compounded with her own insecurities. It didn't happen in a day or even a month. But over time and with iterative practice, Singita grew strong enough to banish the lie. She still must wrestle it to the ground when it comes slinking back unnoticed.

The Takeaway

Too often when we are called to fill the void of another's unexplained intentions, we immediately migrate toward the negative. Then we use our internal dialogue to give the negative statements life and breath.

Be kind to yourself if five minutes only presents a centimeter of the tip of an iceberg you didn't even know was there. To catch yourself in negative self-talk, you can take a simple step like wearing a rubber band around your wrist. Snap it each time you hear yourself say something ugly to yourself. Then you must intentionally redirect your thoughts to a positive replacement thought. Consult a professional if necessary to help you uproot the weeds of deep-seated negative thoughts. Sometimes the prisons we construct in our minds are more powerful than any walls outside of ourselves.

My Journal Reflections

Spend at least five minutes in silent meditation first thing each morning for at least five days this week. Return to this meditation as often and for as long as necessary to truly release bitterness and resentment.

Day 1.   I will use the next five minutes to confront my most negative self-talk habit.

Day 2.   Today I learned this about myself:

_____.

Day 3.   My big lie drives these behaviors within me:

_____.

Day 4.   I am holding onto the lie because:

_____.

Day 5.   If I live my truth, my life will change in this way:

_____.

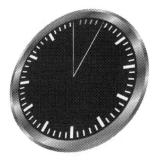

CHAPTER 13

DON'T MIND ALTER

Rashad studied the pills in his hand. They beckoned like whispers in the trees. He didn't want to die, just to sleep for a week. Or maybe until the tension with Bri ended. How long could you sleep with enough dosage and still live? He was so tired of the angry silence that lurked in every room of their home. His anger and desire to leave the marriage were supposed to punish her, but they were choking him. Rolling the pills in his hand, he faced a certain truth: He hated his life.

The Takeaway

Your body is a physical temple in which your consciousness resides. We only get one temple. It is precious and irreplaceable. If injured badly enough, no amount of money can restore it.

In the dark season, it may be tempting to separate your temple from your consciousness. What you are going through might be so painful that this seems like a real option. It is not.

No good comes from taking mind-altering substances that cause you to lose consciousness beyond the kind of assistance that over the counter or medically prescribed medications provide. Leaving your temple unattended can result in many dangerous consequences: Your body may fall into the hands of predators who would harm you; you may be permanently damaged; in a blacked-out state, you may say or do things you'll regret later. Worst of all, you may not be able to wake up. Whatever bad season you are running away from, drinking, or drugging yourself to oblivion is bound to make everything worse. The emotional pain may be excruciating at its peak, but just remember it is darkest before dawn breaks.

Talk to a professional or join a support group if you need to. Persevere. Choose to endure your season of tribulation with your consciousness intact. Yes, you can do it!

My Journal Reflections

Spend at least five minutes in silent meditation first thing each morning for at least five days this week. Resist mind-altering substances as much as possible. Seek professional help if you need it.

Day 1.   My life feels so terrible that I would like to sleep through the next year or so. But I'll take the next five minutes to consider these negative consequences: _____.

Day 2.   I am tempted to leave my temple because:

_____.

Day 3.   I will seek help in coping from:

_____.

Day 4.   I will commit to keeping my mind and body together because I realize: _____.

Day 5.   I will take these steps to help me get through this dark season: _____.

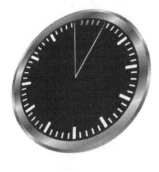

CHAPTER 14

ACKNOWLEDGE HURT

Rashad ultimately decided against the pills. But he still had to sort through his anger and resentment toward Bri. During his meditation time, he worked on the assignment Cassie had given the class. "An early step in the journey to healing is acknowledging the hurt you suffered. Sometimes we carry it around, nurse it, allow it to take over parts of our lives without ever truly expressing it. Sometimes we don't want to let it go," she'd said.

He started with five minutes in the morning but found himself ruminating on the topic throughout the day. Rashad knew he had to face the reasons he was holding on to his anger. Over time, he uncovered several reasons. Only his ability to view them honestly and without judgment allowed him to fully acknowledge them. He was afraid that letting his anger go would condone Bri's hurtful behavior. His anger created a protective shell around his heart. Relinquishing it would open him up to old hurts. He enjoyed treating Bri as if he didn't need her; it made him feel powerful. He also liked being the victim, the wronged. His bitterness was revenge. He didn't know who he would be without his resentment. Letting it go might signal the true end of their relationship.

The Takeaway

Whatever your reasons, it can take a very long time to even acknowledge the depth of pain you have suffered. Today's reflection is just a first step. It might take years to heal, but start by fully acknowledging the hurt that was done to you.

If you have been carrying the hurt around for decades, mentally go back to the age you were when the hurt happened and address the hurt that child experienced.

My Journal Reflections

Spend at least five minutes in silent meditation first thing each morning for at least five days this week. This chapter can take hours and years to unpack fully. Be patient with yourself and stay with it until you really know in your soul that you have let go of the hurt.

Day 1.   For the next five minutes, I will visualize and acknowledge the hurt from a failed relationship or the loss of someone close to me.

Day 2.   What happened hurt me deeply because:

_____.

ACKNOWLEDGE HURT

Day 3.   I haven't moved past that hurt because:_____.

Day 4.   These are all the ways I felt the pain:

_____.

Day 5.   I will express my pain once and for all by:

_____.

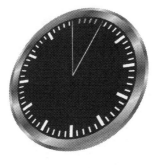

CHAPTER 15

WORRY FAST

Cassie's smile was benevolent. "A worry fast is making the choice to quit worrying cold turkey for some period. Shadow The Cat slid under Singita's dangling feet, enjoying the inadvertent stroking. Singita kicked him in the ribs, making him hiss and flash his one good eye angrily at her before slinking off. Brianna suppressed a grin while Barry scowled. Cassie continued. "Obviously the ideal is that you are on a permanent worry fast. But for most of us, that is very difficult if not impossible to achieve." She let that sink in.

"Fast between certain times. For example, choose not to worry for the first hour of your day. Over lunch, simply enjoy being in the present moment, and don't allow your mind to race." Cassie peered around the room. Shadow The Cat slithered around Rashad's ankles, but he didn't notice. "When you get home at night, decide not to allow that cantankerous spouse or those nagging parents to worry you no matter how vexatious they are." She gestured broadly. "The next day, don't worry about your progress! Just pick up from where you left off yesterday."

The Takeaway

Quelling anxiety is a choice. Your mind won't settle down by itself. You need to *decide* to stop worrying and take active steps to make that happen. The power is yours. Identifying what aspects of a problem you can control may reveal that there's nothing about it that you can, in fact, control. If you cannot control the problem, decide to stop worrying about it because your worry won't change the outcome. And don't worry if this doesn't work the first time you try. As long as there is breath in your body, there is another opportunity to try.

My Journal Reflections

Spend at least five minutes in silent meditation first thing each morning for at least five days this week. Use these topics and your journal to guide your thoughts.

Day 1.   For the next five minutes, I will mentally prepare myself to go on a worry fast for one hour after my meditation.

Day 2.   I am anxious about:

_____.

Day 3. My biggest fear about my problem is:

_____.

Day 4. The worst that can happen is:

_____.

Day 5. Here is what I can control:

_____.

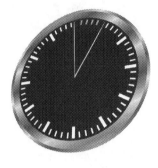

CHAPTER 16

PRACTICE FORGIVENESS

"This forgiveness thing takes forever," Barry said, chugging his black coffee after their workout.

Rashad took a sip of water. "I hear you, man. Every day I spend my meditation time fighting to forgive her. I want to be angry."

Barry nodded. "I get it," he said. He looked around Rashad's pale-green man cave. The swanky shed was lined with shelves boasting obsessively tidy rows of more computer gadgetry than Barry could name. Rashad, a software engineer, had found ways to fill all the time his wife left over the years.

"Holdin' that anger will lead you down my road. In my case, it was my father-in-law's anger but same difference; I'm divorced from the love of my life, drownin' in child support, missin' my kids like crazy, and wonderin' why all our friends went with her."

Rashad studied Barry and then said, "Our kids are in college so …"

Barry waved, dismissively. "Right. But the rest is true. Divorce is awful. You don't wanna go there."

"But you're free! All options open." Rashad was envious.

"To do what, Rashad?" Barry asked. "Go partyin'? Sleep around? Start drinkin' again? Do you really want that life?" Rashad couldn't relate to the drinking part, but he shook his head as he considered.

Barry said, "Decide if you want your marriage and then stay or go. But don't do this." Barry waved figure eights at his friend.

The Takeaway

Barry's is a cautionary tale. Avoid the hard road if possible. It might take years of repeated practice to fully forgive. It's hard.

Forgiveness isn't condoning the other's behavior. It's unshackling yourself so you can move forward.

"Harboring bitterness is like drinking poison
and waiting for the other person to die."

Decide today not to allow your past to hold your future prisoner.

My Journal Reflections

Spend at least five minutes in silent meditation first thing each morning for at least five days this week. This one isn't easy; it's hard. Keep at it.

PRACTICE FORGIVENESS

Day 1. For the next five minutes, I will honestly examine all the reasons I am holding on to my pain.

Day 2. I recognize my negativity hurt me in the following ways: _____.

Day 3. I recognize my negativity hurt people around me in the following ways: _____.

Day 4. I will take these steps to let go of my pain: _____.

Day 5. I wish the one I lost or the one who hurt me well. I will really try to mean it because: _____.

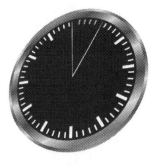

CHAPTER 17

OVERCOME LOSS

"So, what's the story with your dad?" Brianna asked Singita as they left a session. Singita was a petite bouncing splash of red and yellow next to her statuesque companion gliding in muted shades of gold and orange.

Singita sighed. "Appä beat us all except for my youngest sister, Bhakti. My sisters resent her for that." Singita explained her dad's demands for more money than she made, "He thinks that since I live in America, I must be rich." She cackled derisively. After she failed to pay him, refused to marry the stranger who was the son of a great Indian family, and his immigration application was denied, her dad declared Singita dead to him. "He even had a funeral at home in India, so we can never reconcile. And he still uses Ammä to ask for money." Singita hung her head, filled with regrets.

"You need to do what I need to do, Singita," Brianna said. "Accept what's gone. Stop chasing after what you don't have and what you lost. Make peace with it. Accept your past and the fact that your dad could not have been any different. Then inventory what you do have and move forward in appreciation of that."

The Takeaway

Studies have shown that human beings are often more motivated by loss than by what can be gained or even what they have. Singita flowed in the river of negativity that her father created for them both. Even though she couldn't change his ways, she still felt regret and guilt. This relationship influences how Singita treats and views relationships in every aspect of her life. She mourns not just for the father she has but for the one she wishes she had. Acceptance and forgiveness are key parts of healing these kinds of rifts.

My Journal Reflections

Spend at least five minutes in silent meditation first thing each morning for at least five days this week. Your journal may be especially helpful in charting your plan.

Day 1.   I will take the next five minutes to inventory what I have and be grateful for it.

Day 2.   Until today I have been mourning the loss of:

_____.

Day 3.   Until today I have been coveting:

_____.

Day 4.   I have been focused on my lack at the expense of what I do
have, which is: _____.

Day 5.   Going forward, I will focus on what I have because I
know: _____.

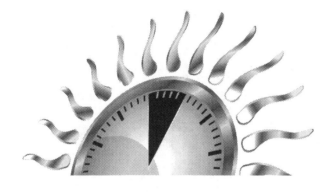

DAWN

The Significance of Dawn

I rise to the brilliant sun beyond the dark ravine.

Dawn is a season of new beginnings:

- A new job, new school, new town you just settled in.
- A new baby or family member.
- A new day full of possibilities.
- The beginning of a new week.

Maximizing your success in this season of newness includes mindfully planning for new opportunities with hope and optimism.

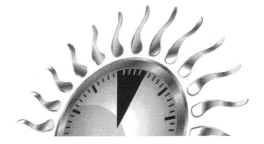

CHAPTER 1

DON'T PANIC

Singita Patel is late! She is watching her sister's three kids for the week while Salma and her husband are on vacation. She leaps from bed and flies around the house like a rogue basketball player with spiked platform stilts and a frenetic ponytail. She rounds up kids, backpacks, and lunchboxes. No bread means she can't make sandwiches. The kids have only one gear—tortoise—so they lollygag.

"I need $20 for today's field trip," chirps her nephew as she screeches into the school parking lot. She has no cash. And her day is just beginning. Aaaaarrrrrrgggggghhhhh!

Across town, Barry Miles is also running late. He calmly trims his red buzz cut. Then he takes five minutes to sit down in his meditation chair and calm himself. He accepts he is running late and can't reclaim that time. During his five minutes, he mentally maps out what he needs

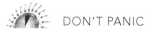

to do to adjust. The last time he didn't take time for himself, he passed out on a plane and almost lost five-year-old Navesh, who was rescued by another passenger. The flight landed safely, but it was a frightening wake-up call. Now, in his five minutes of reflection, he even considers what to say to his tortoises, Naveen and Navesh, to motivate them to crawl faster.

Once on the road, he silently curses the traffic jam, so his chirpy sons don't hear. Even then, he mentally reroutes his day to accommodate the additional delay.

The Takeaway

We all have hectic days. It is counterintuitive to take five extra minutes when you're already behind. Panicking won't help but taking five minutes to collect yourself will. Each time you face a situation you can't control, first pause, and take a calming breath. Acknowledge what you can't control and then adapt to the situation.

My Journal Reflections

Spend at least five minutes in silent meditation first thing each morning for at least five days this week. Consider how you will interrupt your frenetic pace to take five short minutes for yourself no matter how your day begins.

Day 1. For the next five minutes, I will visualize what this day would look like if I floated calmly through every unforeseen upset, no matter how vexing.

Day 2.   My life feels most out of control when:

_____.

Day 3.   My most challenging day of the week is:

_____.

Day 4.   That day is hardest because:

_____.

Day 5.   My new routine first thing in the morning looks like this:

_____.

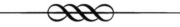

CHAPTER 2

CHOOSE DAWN

"Today we are going to choose our dawn." Cassie smoothed her mud-brown skirt and surveyed the group.

"What d'ya mean?" asked Barry, his gray eyes clouding with suspicion. He cuddled Shadow The Cat in a burly embrace, vigorously scratching his good ear, while the cat seemed to contemplate whether to stay or escape.

Cassie gestured toward him. Her posture and movement made him think of a princess turned hunched young witch. Except during meditation, she always seemed to fold in on herself to be smaller. She said, "Well you're a perfect example, Barry. You're divorced now, right?"

He shifted. "Well yeah," he said. "But you said it could take the next five years to recover from my ten-year marriage."

Cassie nodded. "That's true. But now you can live your dawns. You're not going to be well in a flash; it's an iterative process."

Cassie turned to Rashad and Brianna. "Your children are gone. Time has thrust dawn upon you, but it's up to you to make it wonderful." The couple looked at each other dubiously. "Or you can choose to remain in the dark season. The choice is yours."

The Takeaway

Although dawn can break in your life with a big life-changing event like a new baby, a new spouse, a new home, or a new job, it can also creep in like the sunrise. When it comes, you can choose to bound out of bed and bask in the glow of the rising sun, or you can dive into the dark under your blankets and hide from the glorious rays.

Dawn can be triggered by an event. But more often, it can be a choice. No matter what has happened in your life today, you can choose dawn.

My Journal Reflections

Spend at least five minutes in silent meditation first thing each morning for at least five days this week. Even if your season doesn't feel fully like dawn, consider whether you can choose dawn today.

Day 1.   I will take the next five minutes to examine my life and see what can trigger my dawn.

Day 2.   Today I am choosing my dawn in this aspect of my life: _____.

Day 3.   My dawn has been triggered by this significant life event: _____.

Day 4.   I make the intentional choice not to retreat into the dark season because I recognize: _____.

Day 5.   I will endeavor to stay in my dawn and progress today by making these choices: _____.

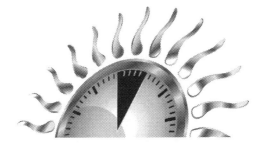

CHAPTER 3

YOUR TRUE DESIRE

"I see you struggling, Bri. Talk to me." Cassie and Brianna sat together after the group session. Cassie noticed that she and Rashad arrived separately from work and didn't go home together.

Brianna patted her hair bun absently. "I don't know, Cassie. I love Rashad. I really do, but …" She trailed off.

"But you're not excited about him, and you know you should be?" Cassie suggested.

Brianna nodded miserably. Her dawn wasn't filled with sunflowers and blue skies.

"Try this. When you do your meditation, first, without judgment, ask yourself what you really want. Just let the answers flow. Don't focus on Rashad. Just in general, what do you want for you?" Brianna nodded.

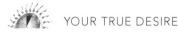

"Accept that every thought you've catalogued doesn't necessarily come from your soul consciousness, your higher self. Your higher self can control your thoughts, but thoughts can be embedded by suggestion and suggested by others." Brianna nodded.

The Takeaway

Strengthening your ability to separate and discern thoughts, sensations, and emotions from your consciousness is the first step to true awareness. Harnessing this power enables you to control yourself and define the direction you really want your life to go. Separating you from your thoughts, sensations, and emotions means you don't have to accept every thought you have as truth. This is especially important in dealing with negative thoughts about yourself and others. Brianna doesn't have to accept as truth everything she thinks about Rashad and their relationship. She can choose which thoughts to reject depending on her desired outcome.

With this in mind, think about what you really want. What do you want that transcends the bonds of materiality? What do you really want that is for your highest and best good?

My Journal Reflections

Spend at least five minutes in silent meditation first thing each morning for at least five days this week. Clarifying your true desire may be harder than you think.

Day 1. For the next five minutes, I will go deep to find the real answer to the question, what do I really want?

Day 2.   I see evidence of my higher self in this way:

_____.

Day 3.   If I set aside materiality, here's what I really want:

_____.

Day 4.   Here's what I want for others close to me:

_____.

Day 5.   Here's what I want for my community:

_____.

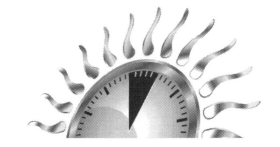

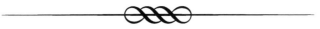

CHAPTER 4

ADDRESS NAYSAYERS

"I want to be a lawyer," Singita blurted out. It was Sunday evening, and four pairs of eyes blinked from her computer screen in stunned silence. Then her eldest sister, Sarani, cackled, exposing the remains of the muffin she was eating.

"You? A lawyer?"

"Reading eight hundred pages of *Anna Karenina* doesn't make you smart," Salma chimed in, completing Sarani's thought.

Singita's bright eyes dimmed, but she looked defiant. "It was 864," she mumbled. Then with a burst of passion she told her sisters about Barry, the lawyer in her support group whose work seemed so fulfilling.

"How will you tell Ammä you're not a doctor?" Sarani demanded. Singita had intentionally emphasized the word physician when she told her parents she was a physician payment and practice management specialist, and they immediately told all their friends their daughter was a rich doctor. While they disapproved of the deception, the sisters kept Singita's secret.

"And law school is so expensive, Singita," said Salma in placating tones. "How will you pay for it?"

The Takeaway

As in Singita's case, sometimes the people closest to us are the ones who hurt us the most. Many motivational speakers advise that if you are embarking on a bold new venture, be careful who you share your dreams with because not everyone will cheer for you, not even your family. When naysayers surface, if their feedback is true and constructive, keep it. Otherwise, bear this in mind:

- No one can define you or hurt you without your permission.
- The most important opinion you will ever have is yours.
- Leave the burden where you found it. Often when people demean and belittle, it's more about them than it is about you. Do not accept that burden and carry it for them.

My Journal Reflections

Spend at least five minutes in silent meditation first thing each morning for at least five days this week. Throw off the cloak of insecurity today!

Day 1. For the next five minutes, I will reflect on constructive feedback I have received without judgment. I will determine how much is accurate and how much is untrue.

Day 2. I believe this information is untrue and borne of these motivations in the person or people who gave it:

_____.

Day 3. Given the naysayers' feedback, I will take the following actions to address it but stay on my current path:

_____.

Day 4. I believe this feedback I received is accurate because:

_____.

Day 5. I will act on the constructive feedback I have received by:

_____.

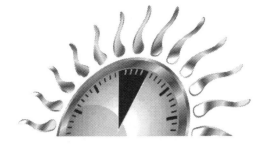

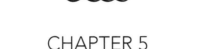

CHAPTER 5
BE ENOUGH

The morning after her jarring conversation with her sisters, Singita sat on her meditation pillow and considered Sarani's ugly words. She remembered all the times during their childhood when Sarani belittled her. She remembered her father's beatings, both with his fists and his words. Only their brother, Bhavin, and youngest sister, Bhakti, were spared. Bhavin because he was a boy, and Bhakti because Appä said she was too black to touch. Singita suspected even he could see that Bhakti was also the most beautiful.

Singita closed her eyes and visualized herself as a lawyer. There she was in a bright red suit, spiked stilettos, a leopard-skin satchel across her back, and striding confidently. She saw the sights, sounds, smells, and tasted what her new professional life would be like. Her current job had a stretched-out title that made her parents think she was important,

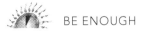

that made her feel important. But being a lawyer would provide real fulfillment.

"I am enough." If she could be a physician payment and practice management specialist, she could be a lawyer.

The Takeaway

Dislodging negative thoughts and self-perceptions so that you can fully step into the dawn of your new opportunities can take a long time. Be patient with yourself. You might have to repeat Singita's week for years, but with consistent practice, it will become easier to see yourself in the new desired light.

As did Singita, examine the motivations of the people who give you feedback in addition to the quality of the feedback itself. In doing this, Singita rejected Sarani's words while accepting the validity of Salma's question and developing an action plan to address it. All the while she affirmed her own self-worth. You can do the same.

My Journal Reflections

Spend at least five minutes in silent meditation first thing each morning for at least five days this week. Stand up for yourself even if you feel as if you are alone in your stance.

Day 1.   For the next five minutes, I will chant, "I am enough," and really think about what it means for me to believe it.

Day 2.   In the past I have not believed I was enough because:

_____.

Day 3.   I sometimes feel like an imposter because:

_____.

Day 4.   I know I am enough for every challenge this day brings because: _____.

Day 5.   Inside me are all the tools and knowledge I need to face this day. Here are the ones I expect to use the most:

_____.

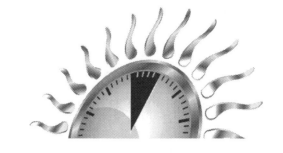

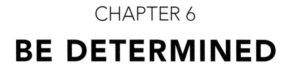

CHAPTER 6

BE DETERMINED

Rashad was determined to have a wonderful evening with his wife when he got home from work. Cassie suggested that enjoying light experiences together might quell his ambivalence about the marriage. He wore the butterscotch-yellow shirt Bri loved because it brought out the glow in his skin. He visualized them talking and laughing about their day. He even meditated on how he'd react if he came home to a cold shoulder. Today he would choose to love her no matter what mood she was in. He even bought her a bouquet.

The moment he walked through the door; he felt the chill. When he saw the sullen look on Brianna's face, he came undone. Like Frosty the Snowman, Rashad's resolve melted away, and he sank back into his old familiar ugly habits of avoidance, deflection, and passive aggressiveness in a sea of stress and resentment.

Too often we give our power away to another to define our state of mind and emotion.

The Takeaway

Without a mature mindfulness meditation practice, most of us are like Rashad. We resolve to change our attitudes, but when challenged, we devolve into old, negative habits.

Dawn is what you make it, and not every day is smooth. You may have to work at it repeatedly to accomplish your goal. Rashad practiced many more evenings before he could stop his mental flowers from withering under the glare of his wife's negative emotions. But with his effort, a strange thing began to happen. She became increasingly pleasant to him.

Part of the benefit of sitting in stillness is recognizing that we are not our emotions. We can observe them and choose not to allow them to drive our behaviors and derail our relationships.

My Journal Reflections

Spend at least five minutes in silent meditation first thing each morning for at least five days this week. Don't be discouraged if your initial efforts to change are unsuccessful. Keep at it.

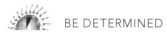

Day 1.   For the next five minutes, I will visualize myself walking through a minefield of turbulence with unyielding calm and serenity.

Day 2.   In the past I have had the most difficulty controlling my emotions when: _____.

Day 3.   I most want to change:

_____.

Day 4.   I will commit to an ongoing mindfulness meditation practice because: _____.

Day 5.   I will not be discouraged if it feels like slow going because:

_____.

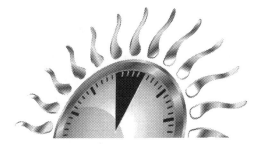

CHAPTER 7

THINK HIGHER

"How did you set aside your issues and move forward in your marriage?" Singita's dark eyes burned with curiosity.

"Well, the issues are still there, but I elevated my thinking," said Brianna. "When I looked at the bigger picture, I realized how petty many of my issues were with Rashad and our marriage." Singita looked skeptical. "Don't get me wrong! I had legitimate issues. But not enough to ditch twenty-three years of marriage. And I still love Rashad."

"So, you just decided to forgive him and be happy and that was that?" Singita looked incredulous.

Brianna laughed. She explained that it wasn't that simple. They were attending marriage counseling to work through all their issues. The bottom line was she had decided to do everything necessary to make it work.

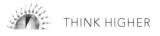

> The Divine: "Well done thou good and faithful servant."
> The Human Soul: "Alas! If I had known this was the game, I would have played with a much better attitude!"

The Takeaway

Brianna's issues with her marriage seemed huge until she put them in a broader context. Your consciousness is greater than the small—in the context of the vast universe—physical temple in which it resides. When you close your eyes for today's meditation, lift yourself out of your body and expand your consciousness. Visualize yourself soaring skyward. Soar into the atmosphere beyond the earth and mentally look down. How big is all that stuff now? Imagine yourself hovering above time. Imagine that you are standing above the span of your life. How important are the day-to-day ups and downs? Will you remember them a year, ten years, fifty years from now?

In your expansive state, where life is the equivalent of a single day when compared to the vastness of eternity, what really matters? How will you wish you had lived this day?

My Journal Reflections

Spend at least five minutes in silent meditation first thing each morning for at least five days this week. Remember that many of the solutions to your life's biggest problems begin with a single decision.

Day 1.   For the next five minutes, I will expand my consciousness beyond the confines of my body.

Day 2.   My biggest challenges right now are:

_____.

Day 3.   Looking down from my higher self, here's what really matters: _____.

Day 4.   Twenty years from now, I will only remember:

_____.

Day 5.   If life is as a single day in the office compared to eternity, here's one thing I'll commit to doing differently:

_____.

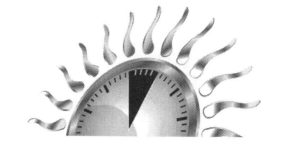

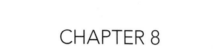

CHAPTER 8

TAME FINANCES

As he settled himself in his meditation chair in a corner of his plush basement, Barry felt peaceful. The four-bedroom house was too big for one. But his father-in-law, Mr. Gupta, had insisted on a home fit for his daughter and grandsons, so he helped Barry with the down payment. Just as Barry's career caught up to his father-in-law's expectations, Mr. Gupta yanked the rug out from under Barry's marriage and persuaded his daughter to return home.

Barry accepted that it might take years to recover fully from his divorce, but his new life was recovering nicely. His finances remained his biggest concern. Better financial habits and a higher-paying job would alleviate the strain. As a new partner at the firm, the pay wasn't yet as good as the title.

Five Things

You can tame finances, no matter your life stage, with these five steps.

1. Identify essential expenses. What's left—your discretionary income—is what you'll use to start your plan for financial freedom.
2. Set aside $1,000 for your emergency fund.
3. Pay off all your debt. Start with the smallest bill and roll that amount over to the next one (debt snowball). Starting with the smallest debt will be rewarding and encouraging when you pay it off.
4. Save three to six months of monthly expenses for your fully funded emergency stash.
5. Out of every paycheck, pay yourself first, and give back by saving at least 10 percent and donating 10 percent.

Automate your plan. Have your paycheck deposited directly into your bank account. Set up automatic payments for everything you can. Automatically transfer 10 percent to your savings and donation accounts. This will increase the chances sticking to your financial plan and freeing up your time.

My Journal Reflections

Spend at least five minutes in silent meditation first thing each morning for at least five days this week. Use the clarity you achieve during your meditation time to chart your financial course.

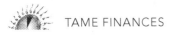

Day 1.   I will take the next five minutes to evaluate my financial situation mentally. No judgment, just the big picture. How happy am I with my current financial situation?

Day 2.   Financial success looks like (Be specific—in success, where you live, how it feels, smells, and sounds like):

_____.

Day 3.   My most significant financial stressors are because:

_____.

Day 4.   The financial decisions I am happiest with or most proud of are:

_____.

Day 5.   My high-level action plan to address my most significant financial concerns looks like this:

_____.

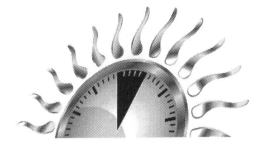

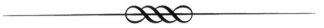

CHAPTER 9

CHOOSE JOY: PART 1

"Share a time that brought you joy," Cassie said. Twelve voices erupted.

"I got a *Gray's Anatomy* science book," Singita chirped immediately.

"Took my sons to a baseball game," Barry said, beaming.

"I came to the States from England," said Fiona Darby.

"Our wedding," said Gene and Jillian Adams in unison.

Each member of the group recounted a joyous event. Then Cassie asked, "How did that make you feel?" The group agreed their joy increased. But then they went back to feeling the way they always felt because the giddiness wasn't permanent.

"Now think of a time when something really bad happened in your life." The answers flew out. Expulsion, a lost job, death of a loved one, a bad diagnosis. "How did that make you feel?" Cassie asked. "Your joy tanked, right? Then what happened? You went back to feeling the way

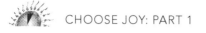

you always felt because that depression—even if it lasted for years or returned periodically—wasn't permanent."

"Prolonged joy can be attained by going within."

Barry shook his head as if trying to dislodge cobwebs. "But what about those people who seem to be annoyingly happy all the time, even when you know they're goin' through trials?" Barry cast a sidelong glance at Singita. She bared her teeth. Barry scowled and looked away.

Brianna missed the exchange. She chimed in, "I know, right? Like that friend who keeps posting about her happy family even though you know her middle child is the product of an adulterous relationship her husband had with another woman."

"Or that buddy who goes on to anyone who will listen about how much he adores his wife even though she just left him," Nandi Chaya said. Barry turned sharply, his freckled face reddening.

"How do they do it? Are they faking it?" Singita wanted to know.

My Journal Reflections

You don't need to fake your joy. Feel it for real and cultivate it daily. Spend at least five minutes in silent meditation first thing each morning for at least five days this week. Dwell with delight on the sources of your joy.

Day 1.   I will take the next five minutes to think about one thing that really gives me joy.

Day 2.   My happiness increased that time when _____ and it
lasted _____.

Day 3.   I sank into depression when:

_____.

Day 4.   My depression lasted:

_____.

Day 5.   I now know permanent joy doesn't come from external,
material things because: _____.

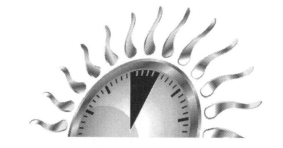

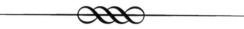

CHAPTER 10

CHOOSE JOY: PART 2

"Maybe some people are faking it, but others have likely discovered a secret about joy," Cassie said, crossing her legs and intertwining her ankles like the rod of Aesculapius, "It's not defined by what's happening out there but by what's going on between your ears." Skepticism colored many of her students. "Studies show that meditation reduces stress, increases the sense of well-being, improves relationships, increases creativity, improves cardiovascular health, enhances the immune system, and can increase your ambient level of joy from within."

Some of the confusion seemed to be clearing. Cassie pushed up her glasses with her middle finger. Barry guffawed. Ignoring him, she pressed on. "Our internal joy is like a thermostat. When something good happens to us, our joy temperature increases but later goes back to its set level. Likewise, when something bad happens, our joy temperature plummets, and we fall into unhappiness or depression. But ultimately, we again return to our set level of joy. It's why you can have a brand-new car, new child, new job, new spouse, and still go back to feeling unhappy or lonely or bored."

"I think I get it," Singita said, her ponytail bobbing vigorously as she nodded. "Sometimes we assume our unhappiness is because something changed in the nature of the spouse, job, or child. But the most likely explanation is that the primary change occurred in us."

The Takeaway

Despite external events, you can achieve and maintain joy no matter what life brings.

"What you seek you will find."

If you focus on the good, the clean, the positive, you will steadily see an increase of that in your life. Over time, and with persistent mindful practice, you can increase your set level of joy by going within and tapping into your personal joy reservoir.

My Journal Reflections

Spend at least five minutes in silent meditation first thing each morning for at least five days this week. Cultivate internal peace and joy during your meditation. Then practice holding on to it for longer periods throughout the day.

Day 1.   For the next five minutes, I will look within myself for peace, contentment, and joy no matter the current condition of my life. I know it's there if I dig deep enough.

Day 2.   The time I tried to use material things to increase my joy went like this: _____.

Day 3.   I see material things haven't brought me lasting joy in that: _____.

Day 4.   I want to increase my joy because: _____.

Day 5.   I will take these steps to go within and tap into the fountain of joy within me: _____.

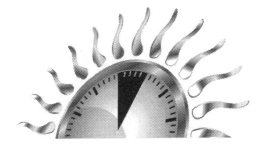

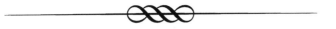

CHAPTER 11

NEVER CRY IN COURT

"He was so mad! He yelled at me the minute the jury left the courtroom," Heather sobbed to her boss, Barry, later. Barry was a partner at a prestigious law firm, and this was his associate, Heather's, first jury trial. As she sat curled in a mousy ball in the large chair in his expansive office, Barry could see that even with his awesome tutelage, she felt outgunned today. Her witness was unavailable for health reasons, and Heather blurted this out in open court rather than seeking a sidebar between the judge and the lawyers. The judge assumed manipulative intent.

Barry listened to her tale of embarrassment at being castigated by the judge in front of opposing counsel. When Heather finished, Barry asked, "Did you cry in court?" Heather shook her head.

Barry leaned forward, resting his elbows on his desk, "So what did you do?"

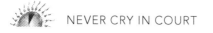

Heather blew her nose. "I stood there and took it. The judge was so disgusted he adjourned for the day, and I left without a word."

Barry leaned precariously back in his chair. Lacing his fingers behind his head, he grinned. "Well done!" he bellowed, making Heather jump. Clearly this was not the reaction she expected.

The Takeaway

Most professionals have had Heather's experience, a gaffe is called out in the most public and shameful way possible. You want to disintegrate on the spot.

"Failure is an occurrence, not a person. Leave yesterday's event where it belongs—in yesterday."

If you are still reliving your mistake from the past, let it go today. You cannot change it. You can only learn from it. But most important, do everything you can not to give it the power to ruin any other day in your career.

My Journal Reflections

Spend at least five minutes in silent meditation first thing each morning for at least five days this week. Focus on clearing your mental decks of negative past experiences and moving forward, free.

Day 1.   For the next five minutes, I will examine a failure I have been carrying around and consciously let it go.

Day 2.   I have been carrying around the memory of that one failure because: _____.

Day 3.   Because I haven't let it go, I have allowed the memory of that one event to limit me in the following ways:

_____.

Day 4.   Today I choose to no longer be held hostage by that one event because: _____.

Day 5.   Going forward, I give myself permission to live and work free of that one incident by: _____.

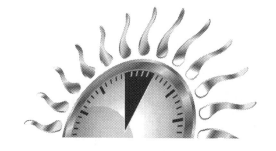

CHAPTER 12

USE FAILURE

Singita aced her first practice bar exam test, just as she expected. But as she regarded her score, she couldn't help wondering why she was such a failure at the relationship with Appä and why her mother always took his side over hers, even when she knew he was wrong.

Across town, Barry pondered his failed marriage and tried to shake the self-blame. He had done everything he could think of to delight his wife—weekly flowers, dinners out. He even massaged her feet when she came home from work. He was devastated when she told him she needed her family and wanted a divorce.

The Takeaway

Sometimes you do everything correctly and still get the wrong result. In those situations, it's easy to become discouraged. You start thinking you're not good enough. You might even believe that the kind of success or happiness you seek is not meant for you. Is there any point in trying?

> Many people find that life is always a little bit crooked in one aspect or another. Sometimes it's a lot crooked.

When people fail at something, too often they define themselves with that event: I failed at this thing, therefore, I am a failure. Or I received a failing grade, therefore, I am not bright. Not only is this false, but it is also debilitating and marks the beginning of your internal negative voice's efforts to derail your motivation, morale, and future prospects.

Understand that life events that appear to be failures are often nothing more than course corrections. Country singer Garth Brooks once talked about the blessing of unanswered prayers because when you're older and wiser, you may find yourself deeply grateful for all the things you desperately wanted but did not receive.

Today accept the wisdom and learning of failed attempts.

My Journal Reflections

Spend at least five minutes in silent meditation first thing each morning for at least five days this week. Be intentional about dislodging negative labels you or others have pasted on your soul.

Day 1.   For the next five minutes, I will express gratitude for my biggest failure. Yes, I will!

Day 2.   Here was a time when something that seemed bad turned out to be beneficial: _____.

Day 3.   Here was a situation I thought was great that turned out to contain negative elements: _____.

Day 4.   In my life today this thing looks bad, but I can see how good may come from it: _____.

Day 5.   I resolve to be more accepting of events that happen in my life by: _____.

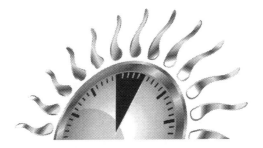

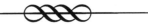

CHAPTER 13

STAY FOCUSED

Brianna was excited. The next day she would give a keynote address for her favorite foundation in front of a thousand people. But she had problems. After a delayed flight from Minneapolis and snarled Chicago traffic, she finally reached the hotel to practice her speech. But setup was in full force in the ballroom where the gala would be held. Workers milled everywhere, rolling banquet tables into place, unfurling table linens, and laying electrical cables that snaked all over the floor.

Brianna's trip to the stage was blocked by a man rolling a table into position. Crew members nearly clobbered her with a projector. She had to wait for a man laying cable to secure it to the floor. The relentless activity thwarted her efforts to reach the stage.

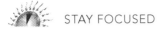

Five Things

You may experience Brianna's day in various ways. Calls, family members, and pets interrupt your workday. A virus cuts into your travel plans and workout routine.

Focus allows you to hold on to your original intention. Allow no distraction to divert your personal, professional, and other goals.

Try these five steps:

1. Get enough sleep. You may need to fight daily to maintain this discipline.
2. Create a consistent daily schedule.
3. Identify your biggest daily distractions.
4. Insert hurdles between you and your distractions. For example, work in a room with no TV, delete social media accounts, or designate after-hours time slots to catch up.
5. Reward yourself for accomplishing each intended task. Take a walk or mindful break, put that load of laundry in. Time yourself so you stay on track.

As for Brianna, despite stubbed toes and irritated workers, she finally reached the podium and practiced her speech to a group of disinterested workers. Her efforts yielded a standing ovation the next day.

My Journal Reflections

Spend at least five minutes in silent meditation first thing each morning for at least five days this week. Like most worthwhile habits, focus doesn't just happen; it must be cultivated and given space to grow.

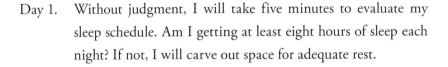

Day 1. Without judgment, I will take five minutes to evaluate my sleep schedule. Am I getting at least eight hours of sleep each night? If not, I will carve out space for adequate rest.

Day 2. My best schedule based on my circadian rhythms and what I want to accomplish today looks like this: _____.

Day 3. My biggest daily distractions are:

_____.

Day 4. Here is my plan for taming distractions:

_____.

Day 5. I will reward myself today for staying on track with my intended tasks.

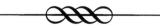

CHAPTER 14

YOU CAN DO THIS

"I don't know how long I can do this, Singi. I feel like I'm failing at everything. The kids don't behave, the house is always a mess, Jopi is always gone, and my best friend is a parrot, literally."

Singita basked in the sun on her patio. Sameena was her closest sibling. While she felt her despair, Singita wasn't discouraged by it. She adjusted her giant multicolored floppy hat to better shield her smooth, honey-toned face from the sun.

"Your best friend isn't a parrot. It's your sister. The kids are wonderful, and your idea of a messy house is a cushion that's not propped the right way," she said.

Sameena tried to smile. Singita told her about her journey through her dark season, the peace she finally made with their appä, and how mindfulness brought her through. She even confided about her law school application. "You are not alone, Sameena. You can do this."

The Takeaway

No matter where you are in life, your self-perception is often different from how others see you. Sameena is successfully raising two wonderful children and holding down the fort. But all she sees is failure. No matter where you are, strive to move forward, but be kind to yourself.

And like Singita, no matter what season you are in, you will be surrounded by friends and family in different seasons. Don't sprint alone. Take time to share your journey with those you trust. If you take time to replenish yourself with the tools of self-care you have found effective, you can give away your love daily and never run dry. Pay attention to those around you who need help.

"Sometimes the circumstances we find ourselves in are just a path to love those we find there."

My Journal Reflections

Spend at least five minutes in silent meditation first thing each morning for at least five days this week. Use a simple mantra like, "I've got this," to encourage yourself in your endeavors.

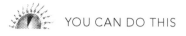

Day 1.   I will take five minutes to identify the aspects of my life I consider the most challenging. I will not judge or become emotionally distraught. Just examine them.

Day 2.   If I put myself in the shoes of someone I know loves me and see myself addressing my challenges from their vantage point, this person would say this to encourage me: _____.

Day 3.   Here are the aspects of my life I am happiest about in this season: _____.

Day 4.   Here are things I borrow from the happy parts of my life to solve my challenges ("can't" and "impossible" are forbidden words): _____.

Day 5.   I am writing down the name of a friend or family member I can encourage and who needs my help. Here's how I can share my love: _____.

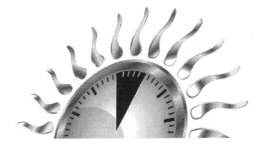

CHAPTER 15

LIVE COURAGEOUSLY

Singita bounced over to her mailbox and froze. There it was. The letter from Harvard Law School. She had secretly dreamed of this letter for years. She had been accepted to other law schools, but this was *the* law school. Since the coronavirus-19 pandemic, all the law schools developed virtual curricula. She couldn't pull this off before, but now she could attend law school anywhere in the country without having to move.

Once in her apartment, her long, orange nails rattled against the counter when she picked up the envelope with trembling hands. It took three tries to slide one talon under the flap. Just as she extracted the letter, her phone rang.

"Are you at home, Singi?" asked Sameena.

The Takeaway

Sometimes we talk ourselves out of opportunities because we are too afraid to even try. We persuade ourselves that our dreams are unattainable. Without judgment or regret, think about the events in your life that have been skewed by fear:

- You passed on a promotion you were qualified for, and then had to train the fool who went for it.
- You clung to a toxic relationship because being lonely was more terrifying than bad.
- You were afraid to speak the truth, and an outcome went sideways.

Not judging includes acceptance.

Accept that you can't change the past no matter how much time you waste looking in the rearview mirror and rewriting things in your head.

Accept that the past could only be what it was because you were who you were, knowing and feeling what you did at that time.

Accept that the only real value the past can have is to inform what you do and who you are now. There is only now.

My Journal Reflections

Spend at least five minutes in silent meditation first thing each morning for at least five days this week. Move into this day boldly no matter what happened yesterday.

Day 1.   I will take the next five minutes to work out in my mind what today will look like if I really live it.

Day 2.   I missed an opportunity out of fear when:

_____.

Day 3.   I held on too long to something out of fear when:

_____.

Day 4.   I don't judge myself because holding on too long had value because it taught me:

_____.

Day 5.   If I really live today, it means:

_____.

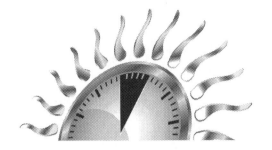

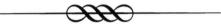

CHAPTER 16

INCREASE FOCUS

Rashad was pleased with the progress he and Bri had made during their dawn season. Each day felt lighter the more he relinquished all the negative feelings he harbored about the marriage.

But he wanted to kick things up a notch at work. Each morning during his reflection time, he wrote down the three most important things he needed to do in order of priority. He scheduled time when he'd check emails, return calls, take a lunch break, and any other interruptions to his day; they ceased to be interruptions when planned. His schedule was constantly derailed by numerous meetings, so he blocked off entire days for back-to-back meetings. Then he blocked off other days when he would not have meetings and just work.

Throughout the day he chose to focus only on the task at hand despite distractions. If someone came into his office, the moment that conversation ended, he turned back to that one thing. He developed a mantra to focus his attention: "This one thing I do."

Five Things

The challenge for most of us is translating vision into reality. Consider using cues that will help keep you on track. For example:

1. Pick the optimum time to wake up, so you can begin each day with the right morning routine.
2. Put your *Mindful in 5* book in your meditation spot, next to your watch or something else you need to start your day.
3. Lay out your clothes if you want to work out in the morning as a visual trigger to start your day the right way.
4. Write down or calendar your tasks if you enjoy checking off lists.
5. Set your *bedtime* alarm so you start preparing for bed and sleep at the optimum time each night.

My Journal Reflections

Spend at least five minutes in silent meditation first thing each morning for at least five days this week. Focus takes practice and time. Keep it up.

Day 1.   For the next five minutes, I will think of the three most important things I must do today and visualize myself in focused execution.

Day 2.   The most important thing I must do today is:

_____.

Day 3.   The second-most important thing I must do today is:

_____.

Day 4.   The third-most important thing I must do today is:

_____.

Day 5.   I will start each day using the following routine:

_____.

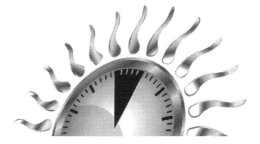

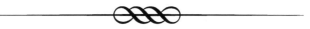

CHAPTER 17

PAUSE ANYWHERE

Singita clicked off her call with Sameena, who waffled but didn't want anything. She was about to return to her Harvard letter when raucous banging erupted at her front door. Letting loose a string of curses in Tamil, her native tongue, she stormed to the door.

"Surprise!" the women yelled. Singita's crimson lips fell open. Her friends, who lived all over the country, were at her door. The group parted to reveal Sameena, holding an envelope high as if it were the Olympic torch.

An hour later, Singita was sitting at a Janet Jackson concert, her favorite artist! Sameena corralled her five friends to celebrate her upcoming birthday. Janet sang a wonderful collection of her new music and old favorites, like "What Have You Done for Me Lately?" and

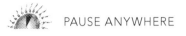

"Escapade." The whole audience stomped around saluting and looking ferocious during the "Rhythm Nation" ensemble.

When she sang the song "Together Again," it was heartfelt and sunny. At the end of the song, the crowd went wild. Janet did something Singita noticed with interest. She stood very still in the middle of the stage. Then she looked up to the heavens, and stretching out a hand, she pointed to the sky. She stood still for a long beat. It was clear she was taking a private moment to commune with someone even with the boisterous horde surrounding her. It was like a calm pool of undisturbed water in the broil of a hurricane. Singita nudged Sameena, and the two stood still amid the roiling, stomping crowd.

The Takeaway

The lesson from Janet's gesture is simple: It doesn't matter what's happening around you. Amid any physical or emotional storm, you can retreat within yourself and connect in a quiet and powerful way. Mindfulness doesn't just work when conditions are optimum. It works all the time.

My Journal Reflections

Spend at least five minutes in silent meditation first thing each morning for at least five days this week. You can be mindfully focused even at the most chaotic time in your day.

Day 1.   For the next five minutes, I will visualize myself taking mindful breaks at intervals during the day, no matter how distracting my surroundings.

Day 2.   My life feels chaotic when:

_____.

Day 3.   I feel like I can't find stillness in my chaotic life because:

_____.

Day 4.   I will take five minutes to be still and breathe when:

_____.

Day 5.   I will take this step to intentionally break from the chaos whenever
my day gets hectic: _____.

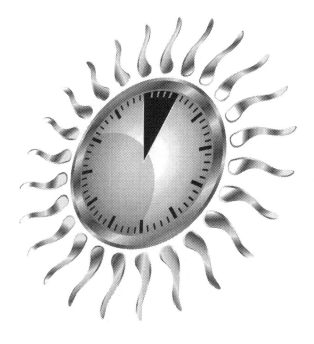

DAY

When Day Breaks, and You Are Loving Life and Living the Dream

During the day season of your life, the sun is shining, and all is well. You are putting one foot in front of the other and living your life. Happiness and even joy come easily. And some people might mistake you for one who is unfairly fortunate.

Here's the secret: The sunshine of your day can last through the dawn and even much of dark. In fact, with consistent mindfulness meditation, you will experience less and less of the dark periods because things that used to plunge you into the abyss of depression and despair are now no more than speed bumps along your life's journey.

Cultivate this sense of peace and calm equilibrium and hold on to it as long as you can. Don't wait to see what the day brings to decide if it's good or bad. Decide it will be a good day at sunrise and hold on to that conviction no matter what each day brings. It might not be smooth all the time, but it will be a lot less bumpy. Fly in the sun of day!

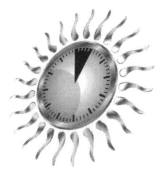

CHAPTER 1

WHY REFLECT?

The twelve watched in fascination as in one fluid movement, Singita folded herself cross-legged into her chair. Not noticing the gawking, she looked balefully around to make sure Shadow The Cat was nowhere nearby.

"I don't know why we're here," Barry Miles threw up his large hands, shattering the spell.

Cassie asked, "How many of you wonder the same thing?" Almost every hand went up. Cassie adjusted her glasses. "When things are going well in life it's easy to abandon practices you adopted when it was hard. But the habits that brought you out of your dark will prolong your stay in the day."

Both Singita and Nandi Chaya leaned in curiously. Gene and Jillian Adams looked perplexed. "How do you mean?" Jillian asked.

"If we continue our mindfulness habits, we are more likely to prolong our season of day and less likely to slip back into dark. Yes?" Brianna asked.

Cassie nodded. "That's right, Bri. It's like filling a reservoir. The more you fill it with thought habits of stability, intentional calm, and presence, the less space the dark days have to take root. So even if you encounter the dark season, it might be less severe, and there will be fewer triggers to shift you back into dark."

The Takeaway

It's easy to cast aside our good habits when things are going well. Once we hit that magic number on the scale, the good eating habits terminate. Once delivered from strife, God-lovers stop praying. Once the thing that had you in the dark season resolves, you skip off into the light without a second thought.

If this describes you, consider this: If your mindfulness meditation habit was strong enough to help you through your dark season, how much more will it help you in the day?

My Journal Reflections

Spend at least five minutes in silent meditation first thing each morning for at least five days this week. Be intentional in committing to your meditation habit in this sunny season.

Day 1.   I will take the next five minutes to give thanks for all the good things that have brought me into this season of day.

Day 2.   To ward against falling off my mindfulness meditation wagon, I will commit to: _____.

Day 3.   Today I commit to my meditation practice during this season of day because: _____.

Day 4.   Today I will center myself in preparation for this day by: _____.

Day 5.   My mindfulness meditation practice can best help me during this happy season by: _____.

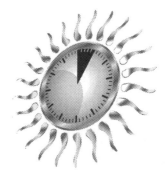

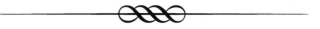

CHAPTER 2
SEIZE THE DAY

"I don't know if this marriage will survive. We're getting along, but I don't know if we'll be together a year from now," Rashad said.

Barry asked, "What would it look like if you stop waitin' for the other shoe to drop? If you stop waitin' for the bad thing to happen?"

Rashad squinted at him, and just then, his phone pinged. He glanced at it and looked perplexed. Barry's brows rose. "My son is trying to solve a problem I can't help with. He's a mechanical engineering major, but I only really know software," Rashad said.

"Ask Cassie," Barry suggested. "She's a mechanical engineer."

"*Mindful in 5* Cassie?" Rashad couldn't conceal his surprise. It was Barry's turn to look surprised.

"Yeah. What do you think she does for a living, counsel schmucks like us all day?" Rashad looked ashamed. He'd never thought about it.

Barry smirked. "Dude, that chick is wicked smart. Refurbishes classic cars and Harleys in her spare time. That's how I met her; we were in the same bike club. I even tried to date her, but she wouldn't have me."

"Cassie?" was all Rashad could manage.

"Open your eyes, man," Barry said. "I bet you don't even know her last name."

The Takeaway

Too many people spend so much time sprinting toward the next thing or gazing in the rearview mirror that they miss what's right in front of them. Yesterday is gone. Tomorrow will tend to itself. There is only now.

Be intentional about luxuriating in what you are doing in the present moment. Psychologists call this savoring. Barry is trying to get Rashad to savor his marriage and the present, regardless of what tomorrow might bring. Rashad's full engagement now may increase the chances that his marriage will survive and even thrive tomorrow.

My Journal Reflections

Spend at least five minutes in silent meditation first thing each morning for at least five days this week. Your life starts now. So, what are you going to do?

Day 1.　For the next five minutes, I will visualize what it will look like if I stop waiting for my life to begin and live it right now.

Day 2.　I have been waiting for this to happen:

　　　　　_____.

Day 3.   I have been discontented with these aspects of my life:

        _____.

Day 4.   Living fully right now means:

        _____.

Day 5.   My decision to start really living today looks like this:

        _____.

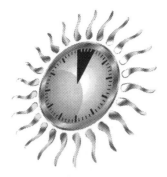

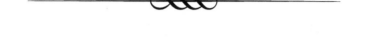

CHAPTER 3

EMBRACE YOUR POWER

"I love my sisters. I do. I just wish they would be more supportive. Especially Sarani." Singita saw empathy brimming in Cassie's green eyes. Shadow The Cat leered at her with his one good eye from beneath Cassie's long brown skirt.

"What's your biggest frustration with this situation?" Cassie asked.

Singita blinked her perfectly made-up smokey eyes. Had she not just said it?

Cassie folded her long, lean frame almost in two as she leaned in to Singita and explained, "Each of us has the unfettered gift of choice. You have no control over the family you were born into, but you have complete control over the choices you make in your life. You can't control how others behave, but you control your own attitudes, behaviors, and reactions.

The Takeaway

Cassie's point applies to all of us. In all areas of life there is a choice of at least two things. For example, if someone maligns you, you have the choice of reacting in kind or not. If you were raised in an environment where certain negative behaviors were the norm (for example, alcoholism, domestic violence), you have the choice of continuing that cycle or not.

This absolute gift of choice carries absolute responsibility. Too often people disclaim the responsibility by saying, "I had no choice." What they really mean is they so disliked the other choice they chose to simply pretend it didn't exist. It is also a way of sidestepping ownership and responsibility for the choices we make.

The absolute gift carries absolute power to control yourself. It doesn't mean the choices will be easy or popular. Some choices you make will have agreeable outcomes, while others yield unintended lifelong consequences. But the fact remains the power to choose is always in your hands.

My Journal Reflections

Spend at least five minutes in silent meditation first thing each morning for at least five days this week. Practice owning your choices without beating yourself up even if you didn't like the consequences.

Day 1.   For the next five minutes, I will contemplate a big choice in my life right now and fully own it.

Day 2.   I have avoided owning this choice in the past:

_____.

Day 3.   I am avoiding owning this choice now:

      _____.

Day 4.   Without judgment, I own that choice. I made it because:

      _____.

Day 5.   Today I will respond this way when something unpleasant
happens: _____.

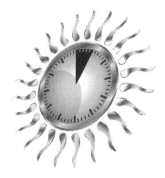

CHAPTER 4

STAND BRAVELY

On the sprawling Lake Forest, Illinois, campus, Bri hopped on the elevator. Her coveted meeting was minutes away. Gottfried Kaufman was CEO of Sunderland Medical, subsidiary of a global conglomerate on par with Google and Amazon. He was so impressed with a speech she gave at a foundation dinner that he invited her for this meeting. Brianna was the only Black person and the only woman on the elevator. The white men were dressed in dockers, white shirts, and dark blazers. Her dark blazer covered a tasteful African-print dress and matching jewelry she had purposefully chosen. With her lithe body, long graceful neck, and bun topped with a cascading crown of natural curls, she looked regal. She had never fit in and never would, so there was no sense in hiding. She smiled. *All the better to be memorable, my dear*, she thought.

The Takeaway

You came into this world as an individual with unique gifts. With those gifts you will serve purposes only you can. No one will lay footsteps in your exact pattern through life, and only you will leave this world at your appointed time.

There is only one you. As social creatures, human beings tend to seek the company of others, and we tend to seek conformity.

If you ever felt different because of your appearance or something you viewed as a peculiarity, you know the discomfort of nonconformity. If you felt at home as one of the men on Bri's elevator, you know the comfort of belonging. In that case, it may sometimes be difficult to be memorable and shake a veneer that might render you invisible.

Embrace yourself and your unique skills, capabilities, and talents. They are yours on purpose, and you are perfect just as you are right now. This is who you are. Rise.

My Journal Reflection

Spend at least five minutes in silent meditation first thing each morning for at least five days this week. Stepping into the power of who you are is not once and done. It is a daily decision, and when you live life intentionally, you will become conscious of the myriad times in a day when you must choose this fork in the road during that meeting, in responding to emails, in the temptation to hide behind the wisdom of others.

Day 1.   I will spend the next five minutes visualizing what it will look like if I truly step into my own voice.

Day 2.   I wished I conformed when:

      _____.

Day 3.   I feel alone because:

      _____.

Day 4.   I embrace the singularity of who I am because I realize:

      _____.

Day 5.   I will learn to love myself by:

      _____.

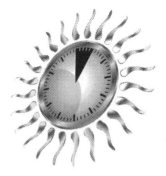

CHAPTER 5

LONELY OPPORTUNITIES

It was Friday night, and Barry was going to miss Bri and Rashad's big bash the next evening. He felt lonely stepping on to the flight from Minneapolis to Chicago on an evening when so many travelers were coming the other way. He received a first-class upgrade, doubtless, he figured, because of his disarming smile and cool kicks. He wore his comfy faded jeans and white T-shirt accentuated by his favorite two-tone Texas state heritage belt. Rockport sandals showed off what he viewed as the sexy red hair on the arcs of his toes.

But he was excited. Barry had an interview for a big job as associate general counsel of Sunderland Medical, subsidiary of the largest manufacturing company in the world.

The Takeaway

Most people don't like lonely opportunities, especially when they are the only ones working when everyone else is having fun. Moreover, you rarely hear anyone talking with glee about being the only woman, the only person of color, or the only white guy in the room.

> Sometimes being lonely is really being
> set apart for your life's purpose.

There was only one Martin Luther King Jr., one Mother Teresa, one Mahatma Gandhi, and one Abraham Lincoln. We are all created in our own significance, so we won't be like any of these individuals. Nonetheless, you hold the power in your hand to change other people's lives for better or worse in ways only you can. The choice is uniquely yours. Decide right now to never again gripe about being "the only." If you feel the pressure to represent your entire demographic, then contribute something meaningful. That way, the next time someone like you walks through the door, he or she might not be disregarded as you were or mistaken for the help.

Embrace the lonely opportunity, and make it count.

My Journal Reflections

Spend at least five minutes in silent meditation first thing each morning for at least five days this week. Embrace the lonely opportunities.

Day 1.   For the next five minutes, I will visualize with gratitude my lonely opportunities.

Day 2.   Here is a time when I was "the only":

_____.

Day 3.   Here's how I felt about it then:

_____.

Day 4.   It was an opportunity in this way:

_____.

Day 5.   Here's how I will embrace future lonely opportunities: _____.

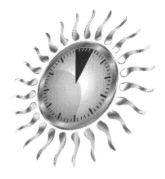

CHAPTER 6

EVALUATE FRIENDSHIPS

"How was your meeting?" Singita asked Brianna. She loved her customary afternoon of crossword puzzles and Sudoku but gladly relinquished them to walk briskly around Lake Harriet on a sunny Saturday afternoon.

Brianna gushed about Gottfried Kaufman. "When I stepped in, he clicked his heels, bowed, kissed my hand, and said, 'Greetings, your highness." Brianna laughed.

Singita frowned. "Really? I heard his employees call him a tyrant."

"Well, he knows how to charm because he was wonderful. He pledged a hefty donation to our school." The two friends chattered on, Singita cheerfully filling the silent spaces between their conversation with happy slurps of her ice-cream cone.

The Takeaway

Friendships are valuable in every setting. Psychological research demonstrates that having a best friend reduces stress. Research also shows that employees are more likely to stay with an employer if they have a best friend at work.

"Try this definition for the next thirty days:
A friend is good to you and good for you."

This is not gospel, but a simple barometer by which to gauge genuine friendships. If someone isn't both things, it might still be a worthwhile relationship, but he or she might just not be your friend. For example, a coach or teacher might be good for you but not necessarily good or even nice to you. A friend who leads you astray may be good to you but not good for you.

You don't need to ditch people who are not true friends. However, awareness of your relationship dynamics allows you to set realistic expectations and be intentional in how you engage, and how much of yourself you give.

Accept people as they are. It's not your place to fix anyone to better suit yourself. Take care of yourself by minding your friendships.

My Journal Reflections

Spend at least five minutes in silent meditation first thing each morning for at least five days this week. Even if you decide someone isn't really your friend, evaluate the value of the relationship. It may lie in a different avenue than you previously thought.

Day 1.   For the next five minutes, I will evaluate my closest relationships.

Day 2.   My three closest friends are:

_____.

Day 3.   The five people most good to me are: _____.

Day 4.   The five people most good for me are:

_____.

Day 5.   I need to change my relationship with _____
because: _____.

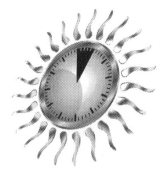

CHAPTER 7

MINDFUL CELEBRATION

Barry sat on a barstool at his sun-drenched kitchen island first thing in the morning. His hands still shook as he read the letter from Sunderland Medical for the hundredth time: "Dear Mr. Miles, we are delighted to offer you the role of associate general counsel." He'd start in two weeks. The benefits package and the job itself were beyond anything he had ever dreamed of. His child support payments would increase, but there would be much more cushion for the rest of the bills. And he could even afford to use his six weeks of vacation doing interesting things with his boys.

What Barry really wanted to do was have a drink and spend the next two weeks leaping for joy. But remembering Cassie's admonition that mindfulness and meditation were especially valuable when the sun shone its brightest, he bounded down to the basement, settled in his meditation chair, rested his forearms on his thighs, and closed his eyes.

He began his *Mindful in 5* meditation by centering himself with breathing exercises. Then he gave thanks for all that he had endured, including the painful end to his marriage and the divorce that brought him to this point and made him all that he had become. Before he knew it, half an hour had gone by. But when he arose, he felt rejuvenated, refreshed, and ready for the day.

The Takeaway

Hopefully your life is filled with many days like this one. Good news abounds, and the sun shines brightly on your future. You can always reflect with gratitude.

No matter what season of life, there are always reasons for gratitude.

On days when all is well, take time to catalog all the things for which you are grateful.

My Journal Reflections

Spend at least five minutes in silent meditation first thing each morning for at least five days this week. Commit to maintaining your habit especially in this season, when it's so easy to abandon your good habits that brought you this far.

Day 1.   I will take the next five minutes to catalog all the reasons I am in my day season.

Day 2.   I am most grateful for this source of joy in my life:

_____.

Day 3.   I am grateful for this second-most significant source of joy in my life: _____.

Day 4.   Here's what I like the least about my season of day, and here's what I can do to turn it around:

_____.

Day 5.   No matter what today brings, I will remain in my season of day, and my day will look like this:

_____.

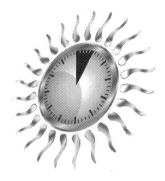

CHAPTER 8

MINDFUL FRIENDSHIPS

"So how are you doing, Barry? What's happening here?" Rashad asked, waving his pool stick around Barry's basement before he took his shot. Rashad came over to play pool a few times a month.

A recovering alcoholic, Barry had no booze in the house, so the two men drank sodas. He ran his large hand across his buzz cut, hair bowing like red grass to a gust of wind. "Actually, I'm doin' great."

"You've come a long way, man. I remember finding you catatonic that day on your couch with the child support notice in your lap."

Barry nodded, "Yep, you kicked my butt." The two men burst into laughter. Rashad had dragged Barry outside with a football and tackled and hit him with it until the two men got a nice game of two-man tag going. Then some neighbors joined in, and the afternoon improved.

Rashad grinned. "And now here you are. And you even got that job at Sunderland!" The two men bumped fists.

The Takeaway

Barry and Rashad exhibit traits of healthy mindful friendships.

1. Consistent connection. Mindful friendships involve consistent contact. It's best if both friends make an effort to connect.
2. Mutual recharging. Creating a safe space to recharge together can go a long way to reducing stress.
3. Mastermind life. A mindful friend can provide helpful insights, ideas, networking contacts, and other resources professionally or personally.
4. Fun memories. Mindful friends can lighten tough situations. And they can laugh about anything—at least in hindsight if not now.

This is not an all-inclusive checklist. Your friendships are not deficient if all these characteristics are not present. But if you take an honest look, you will likely discern whether you have healthy friendships.

My Journal Reflections

Spend at least five minutes in silent meditation first thing each morning for at least five days this week. It's okay if your friendships aren't perfect since neither are you!

MINDFUL FRIENDSHIPS

Day 1.   For the next five minutes, I will think about my three closest
         friends—what they pour into me, and what I pour into them.

Day 2.   My best friendship is with _____
         because: _____.

Day 3.   I am a good friend to _____
         because: _____.

Day 4.   My closest friendships have these characteristics:
         _____.

Day 5.   To be a better friend, I will:
         _____.

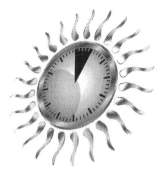

CHAPTER 9

FIVE STRENGTHS

"Did you tell your sisters you got into Harvard Law School?" Brianna asked Singita. Big brown eyes rolled to the sky as Singita's cherry lips quirked at the ends. "So, they still think you're a physician blah, blah, blah?"

"Physician Payment and Practice Management Specialist." Singita rattled off the title with practiced smoothness. When she told her parents, all they heard was physician. They toasted to their impending wealth now that their daughter was a rich doctor. Singita allowed them their misconceptions. When she failed to send thousands of dollars home monthly, Appä hurled insults.

"What are your five greatest strengths, Singita?" Bri interrupted her thoughts.

Singita's brows dropped into a thick line. She couldn't think of five.

The Takeaway

Identifying our strengths can be difficult. We are much quicker to see the positive qualities in others.

This week is all about building yourself up without being egotistical. Examine and embrace your five greatest strengths. Return to this reflection whenever you need to remember the value that lies within you. Remember that five-minute meditations are a jump-start, not a limitation.

Sit for as long as necessary for each strength to really sink in and for you to fully grasp and accept them as your gifts.

You are perfect as you are right now.

If you can't think of five positive things, borrow from positive comments people have made to you and about you, even if you didn't believe them. If you are still stuck, think of a time when someone said something to you like this:

- "You have such a gift of compassion."
- "Gosh, you are so good with children."
- "You're a lifesaver! We couldn't have salvaged that project without you."
- "Thank you for being my friend. I really appreciate you."

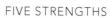

My Journal Reflections

Spend at least five minutes in silent meditation first thing each morning for at least five days this week. Don't be shy; toot your own horn to yourself. You must first appreciate your own value to fully leverage it in the world.

Day 1. I will take the next five minutes to ponder five strengths that I have. I can immerse myself in them without being egotistical.

Day 2. Of my five strengths, my greatest one is:

Day 3. People most often tell me I am best at:

        _____.

Day 4. In the past I have shied away from claiming this power within myself: _____.

Day 5. I need to own my strengths by: _____.

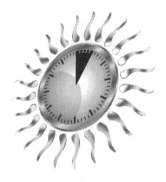

CHAPTER 10

CHOOSE GRATITUDE

"All right everyone," Cassie said, quieting the buzzing circle of twelve. "Let's talk about gratitude."

"Why is gratitude such a big deal?" Barry asked. He rocked precariously on the hind legs of his chair, burly arms crossed, legs sprawled in front, cargo shorts boasting hairy muscled legs.

Cassie picked up a partially toothless yawning Shadow The Cat. "Gratitude isn't just fluffy foolishness practiced by privileged people. According to the article you read for today, gratitude can deliver four major benefits. Who remembers?"

Happy to know where the creepy cat was, Singita chirped, "Stress and pain relief. Gratitude is associated with the same neural networks in the brain that mobilize when we feel pleasure or socialize."

"The same parts of the brain that control certain functions such as heart rate, arousal, pain, and stress reduction," Jillian Adams piped in.

"Excellent," Cassie said.

Fiona Darby added, "Gratitude can lead to health benefits over time because it uses those same neural networks that relieve stress and engage during social bonding."

"Indeed," Cassie agreed, caressing the cat's bony spine.

"Gratitude can also improve sleep, romantic relationships, reduce the likelihood of illness, increase motivation for exercise, and boost happiness," Fiona answered.

Cassie nodded. "What else? There's one more.

"I read one study where practicing gratitude rewired the brain, alleviating depression," Rashad said.

"To some degree, yes." Cassie agreed. At the end of the session, she asked them to list as many things as possible to be grateful for over the next week.

The Takeaway

Let go of the myth that only happy people are grateful for their charmed privileges. Many people are happy—joyful even—because they practice gratitude for all that life brings. Everyone in Cassie's group was struggling with something, yet sources of gratitude could be found.

My Journal Reflections

Spend at least five minutes in silent meditation first thing each morning for at least five days this week. Consider practicing gratitude daily by thinking of a few things each morning you are grateful for even before you get out of bed.

Day 1.   I will take the next five minutes to think about the relationships for which I am most grateful.

Day 2.   I am grateful for the following three blessings in my life: _____.

Day 3.   I am grateful for the following three failed relationships: _____.

Day 4.   I am grateful for the following big disappointments: _____.

Day 5.   I am who I am today because of these high and low experiences: _____.

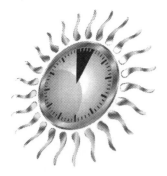

CHAPTER 11

LOVE ANYWAY

Singita beamed at her sisters. Since their last meeting, she had meditated on loving them no matter how they behaved. She visualized herself treating them lovingly. She even visualized her eldest sister, Sarani, reaching through the video chat screen and slapping her hard across the face. In her meditative reverie, Singita's head whipsawed, ponytail flying, and the sting left a red imprint. But she composed herself, smiled at her sister, and said, "I love you, Sarani." She repeated the phrase until she said it with genuine affection no matter what her sister said.

Every day she visualized herself behaving and speaking in a loving manner toward each of her sisters. Some were easier than others.

After all her practice, Singita's days of concentration paid off. She didn't fly off the handle when Sarani made her usual snarky comments. She came to her youngest sister's defense when some of the others poked fun at Bhakti, and she was her usual loving self to her favorite sister, Sameena.

The Takeaway

Too often we think of love as a noun, something we stop doing when we no longer feel it toward an activity we committed to or people around us. In this example, Singita used love as a verb, something she exercised regardless of how she felt.

Acting in love toward others eliminates the excuse of how you feel. You can love your spouse even when you don't feel like it, just as you can love your kids, your relatives, and your friends regardless of how you feel about them. You can even do your job as if you love it even if you don't.

Hold yourself to a higher standard. Adopt love the verb.

My Journal Reflections

Spend at least five minutes in silent meditation first thing each morning for at least five days this week. Don't skip the days that have challenging assignments. Really lean in and tackle those.

Day 1.   I will identify someone challenging to relate to and take the next five minutes to examine my behavior toward him or her the last time we met.

Day 2.   I get along well with _____, and here's how I behave toward them that conveys love: _____.

Day 3.   I find this family member challenging: _____. Behaving in a loving way toward him or her would look like this: _____.

Day 4.   Here's an activity I love and what it looks, feels, tastes, and sounds like: _____.

Day 5.   Here's what my day would look like if I actively loved everything set before me to do:

_____.

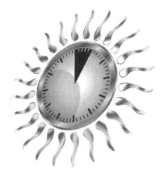

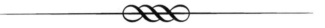

CHAPTER 12
FIND CONTENTMENT

Rashad and Brianna sat cross-legged on their meditation pillows facing each other. Hands resting lightly on their knees, they gazed at each other and smiled. For the first time in a long while, Brianna admired her husband's handsome face and caring eyes.

"Our kids are still gone," Brianna said.

"We are still adjusting," Rashad replied.

"I choose you anyway," said Brianna.

"I love you more every day," Rashad said.

They were on different pages of their *Mindful in 5* book. They read their books in silence and afterward, closed their eyes to meditate on their individual topics.

The Takeaway

Reestablishing an intimate emotional connection with a loved one begins with a choice followed by action. Likewise, falling in love with the life you have right now is a choice. The following five factors can lead to greater fulfillment.

1. Decide to love the life you have right now. Rain falls into every life. Accept that yours is exactly what it should be right now.
2. Eliminate feelings of entitlement. Thoughts like, *I should have,* and *I should be* sow discontentment and frustration.
3. Live in the present. Yesterday is gone and can't be changed. Worrying won't change tomorrow. Enjoy the moment you have right now.
4. Do something nice for someone. Our self-focused society encourages us to always be concerned with our own comfort. Step outside yourself and experience the joy of giving.
5. Set goals and take the first step to achieving that thing you've always wanted to do. Being mindfully present does not absolve you of the need to plan and set goals for your life. Planning also helps you to feel a sense of purpose in where you are going that will hopefully resolve any need to worry about the future.

My Journal Reflections

Spend at least five minutes in silent meditation first thing each morning for at least five days this week. Don't covet another's life or things. Just focus on the blessings and challenges in your own life, remembering that both qualities are necessary for wholeness.

FIND CONTENTMENT

Day 1.   For the next five minutes I will decide to be content right now regardless of how messy my life is.

Day 2.   I worry I am missing out on:

_____.

Day 3.   I see others succeeding and passing me by in these ways:

_____.

Day 4.   Embracing my life as it is right now means accepting:

_____.

Day 5.   Choosing to be content right now means:

_____.

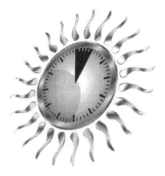

CHAPTER 13

CELEBRATE MILESTONES: PART 1

"Celebrate every milestone, no matter how big or small," Cassie said. Most were too busy studying her to listen. "Barry, what's your milestone?"

Barry the Cheshire exposed all 57 teeth, "My divorce is done, my sons are thriving, and I got this amazing new job!" The group broke into applause.

"I finally did my *Mindful in 5* meditations five consecutive days," said Singita, bangles chiming and ponytail bobbing.

"What about you, Cassie?" asked Rashad, staring at her. Murmurs of agreement followed as twelve pairs of eyes stared. Slowly she rose and pirouetted. Gone were the drab, flannel, shapeless skirts and dresses. They were replaced by a white, low-cut cami shirt and a dark blazer. A bulky necklace showed off her long, slender neck. High-rise skinny jeans accentuated her lean frame. Flesh-colored heels punctuated the ensemble, adding to her height. The pale ginger bush at the nape of her neck was replaced by a trendy, short, vibrant, curly cut complete with fresh highlights. She moved with a dancer's grace that hadn't been there before she began feeling as beautiful on the outside as she felt inside.

Rousing applause.

"You look like a tall, green-eyed Meg Ryan," Barry blurted.

"Don't you need your glasses?" Nandi Chaya asked.

"Contacts." Cassie beamed. Some wanted to know how the transformation happened. "Girls' day out with them," sang Cassie, pointing at Brianna and Singita.

The Takeaway

"If you can first think it, you can do it, and then you can be it."

As with Singita, it might take a lot of mental energy and continued practice to take steps toward your goal. The journey may feel like a slog, not at all sexy or glamorous. But the path to great success is often paved with sweat, doubt, and tears. The outcome, though, can look like Cassie.

My Journal Reflections

Spend at least five minutes in silent meditation first thing each morning for at least five days this week. Use these topics to propel yourself further into your season of day.

Day 1.   For the next five minutes, I will visualize myself doing that thing I long thought impossible.

Day 2.   I have always wanted to:

_____.

Day 3.   To get there, I need to:

_____.

Day 4.   Step one of my goal is to:

_____.

Day 5.   To start moving toward my goal, I will:

_____.

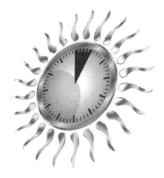

CHAPTER 14

CELEBRATE MILESTONES: PART 2

"I don't have a milestone," Gene Adams said. "My job is my issue. I'm just not fulfilled." Gene rested his elbows on his knees and looked mournful.

Across from him, Barry leaned back and clasped his hands behind his head. "Wantin' too much from the job, dude."

Cassie regarded him with interest. "What do you mean, Barry?"

Barry said, "We expect the job to deliver intrinsic joy, fulfillment, wholeness, wealth." He gestured expansively. "If you get all those things out of your job, great! But that's not why you were hired."

The group explored this idea and left Gene with specific reflections to work on during his meditation time.

The Takeaway

Your employer hired you to solve a problem in exchange for your pay. Not being delirious about the job doesn't make it wrong. Start by being grateful for the job you have. For instance, they pay you. Next, consider all the things you can afford because of it.

There's a story in the Bible about a merchant who hired laborers throughout the day to work for him. At the end of the day, he paid the ones who worked one hour the same as he paid the ones who worked all day. Of course, the ones who worked the longest were angry. Most employees take the perspective of the all-day employee: "I'm overworked, underpaid, and taken advantage of."

But to employers, many employees are like the one-hour laborer— work an hour and expect a whole day's wage! Contentment comes in viewing yourself as the one-hour servant, receiving more than you deserve. After all, you are not entitled to the job you have, and there would be a long line of candidates vying for it if you left.

Journal Reflections

Spend at least five minutes in silent meditation first thing each morning for at least five days this week. Work is a source of dissatisfaction for too many. Confront your real feelings about your job this week.

Day 1. For the next five minutes, I will visualize what it will look like to be my best at work.

Day 2. I am dissatisfied with my job because:

_____.

CELEBRATE MILESTONES: PART 2

Day 3.   My employer hired me because:

_____.

Day 4.   The problem my job addresses is:

_____.

Day 5.   I am grateful for my job because: _____.

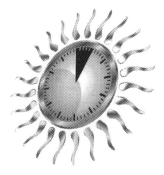

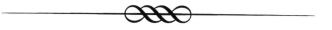

CHAPTER 15

CELEBRATE MILESTONES: PART 3

Cassie listened carefully to Barry's comments to Gene and then chimed in. "Being mindful about the expectations you have of your work helps to identify areas of dissonance between what you expect from the job compared to what the job really is."

Gene nodded, deep in thought.

Cassie continued, "Mindfulness is about observing what's within and around you without judgment. Any divergence between your expectations and the reality of your job is not a point of disappointment or angst. Just see it for what it is."

"Then pivot," Brianna said. "Once you see the job for what it is, waste no time on negative emotion. Look for ways to find meaning in the work that you do."

Gene squinted at her. "What do you mean?"

Brianna thought a moment and then said, "Start by finding the why of the job. Why does your job exist?"

Gene laughed and flapped his hands in surrender. "I'm a janitor at a hospital. Where's the meaning in that?"

Brianna didn't miss a beat. The schoolteacher in her flared. She looked him squarely in the eye and declared in an authoritative tone that made everyone sit up straight, "It is your responsibility to ensure the highest levels of cleanliness and sanitation in that hospital, which contributes to positive health outcomes for patients and ensures the safety of their loved ones who walk the halls every day." Next to Gene, his wife, Jillian, mouthed a silent, *Thank you*, to Brianna.

The Takeaway

Every job exists for a reason. No employer pays good money for no reason. You might be looking for a new job, but while you have this one, find the why. Then lean into that reason and execute with mindful excellence. Easier said than done? Yes. Worth trying? Absolutely.

My Journal Reflections

Spend at least five minutes in silent meditation first thing each morning for at least five days this week. Until you find your next dream job, ignite yourself to do your very best at this one.

Day 1.   For the next five minutes, I will focus on the real reason my job exists. Then I will find a way to light my fire with it.

Day 2.   When I think about it more deeply, my job impacts customers in this way: _____.

Day 3.   On the surface, here's what I do:

_____.

Day 4.   Here's how my performance impacts my employer's business:

_____.

Day 5.   How I do my job impacts my coworkers in the following ways:

_____.

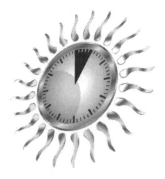

CHAPTER 16

LAST DAY

"I know what it's like to lose your dad," Rashad said. "One day my dad woke up feeling unwell, and within twenty-four hours, he was gone. When he saw death coming, he didn't panic. He arranged his will and his weapons in plain view and prepared. He thought of everything. We had a great relationship, but he didn't call me."

He ducked as Singita kicked up a noisy spray with her legs in the pool at Rashad and Brianna's house, red toenails carving arcs in the air.

Rashad continued, "He didn't need to because we expressed love to each other in every interaction."

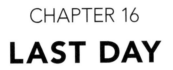

"Live a life of no regrets. Share your love now.
Share your appreciation now. Take that risk now."

"I've made peace with who my appä is," Singita declared, surveying with satisfaction the damp circle she'd created around them that included Rashad's shorts. "To his dying day, he'll be a mean, stingy man who enjoyed beating his daughters until we escaped that mad household."

Rashad's brows shot up. This level of detail was new to him.

"Cassie showed me how to use mindfulness meditation to go into that pain, acknowledge it, fully experience it, and then let it go."

The Takeaway

Rashad and Singita had starkly different experiences with their fathers. Nonetheless, they are both at peace. If this were your last day, what would you wish you had or had not done? Plan to address any outstanding desires now.

My Journal Reflections

Spend at least five minutes in silent meditation first thing each morning for at least five days this week. Hindsight changes perspective. Don't let another day pass without mending a broken relationship you would regret leaving in its current state.

Day 1. For the next five minutes, I will visualize what I would want today to look like if I knew it would be my last.

Day 2. If today were my last day on earth, I would regret not repairing my relationship with: _____.

Day 3. If today were my last day, I would wish I had:

_____.

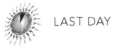

Day 4.   To avoid life's regrets, today I will:

_____.

Day 5.   I will live my life with the following mindset:

_____.

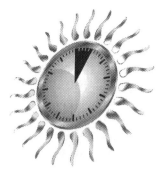

CHAPTER 17

LAST CLASS

"Thank you for attending this group." Cassie's intelligent eyes held their customary compassion as she beamed at the group. "What have you learned?" Singita mumbled something about that scruffy cat. The other eleven were so busy smiling and nodding that no one spoke. "*Bam,*" Cassie yelled, startling them but bringing out all of Barry Andrew Miles's 57 teeth at a hundred watts.

"Well, Cassie, thanks to y'all and my *Mindful in 5* book and practice, I made peace with my divorce. I love my wife, and I hate that she left. But it's all right, and I have really bonded with my boys," Barry said, conjuring Shadow The Cat and stroking him tenderly. The cat vibrated from rumbles of delight.

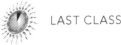

Rashad beamed tenderness at his wife and held out his palm. She clasped it tightly. "It was a long road, but we received many insights during our meditations that led us to recommit to our marriage."

Brianna laughed. "Cassie, you said start with five minutes, but there were times I swear Rashad sat for hours!"

"Grappling with the challenges of life takes time," Cassie said. When the couple invited the group to the ceremony for the renewal of their vows, cheers went up.

Next was Singita. "I finally let go of my issues with Appä. It took a lot of hard work and support from my friends." Singita attempted a smile. It was beautiful, but she always looked awkward when she smiled, as if she didn't grow up doing it. But the class smiled back warmly. "Things are much better between me and my eldest sister, Sarani. She's still a condescending witch, but I accepted her as she is, so she's my condescending witch." Everyone laughed. "Ironically, our getting along better has strengthened the bond between all my sisters, so I'm grateful."

After all had shared, the group departed with hugs and promises to get together socially.

My Journal Reflections

Spend at least five minutes in silent meditation first thing each morning for at least five days this week. Take time to reflect on your mindfulness journey, the discipline you have harnessed, and how you have grown.

Day 1. I will take the next five minutes to reflect on what I've learned through my *Mindful in 5* book and journey.

Day 2. My biggest takeaway from this journey is:

_____.

Day 3.   Through my mindfulness practice, I have learned:

      _____.

Day 4.   I will continue in my mindfulness meditation practice by:

      _____.

Day 5.   I will share *Mindful in 5* with _____, who I know can benefit from it.

EPILOGUE

Akar, VP of sales at Sunderland Medical, raised his glass. Chantelle, the company's chief legal officer, had invited him to meet her friends, Rashad and Brianna, at a party she threw after they renewed their vows. "To weathering work!" Akar cried with aplomb.

"To weathering work," Chantelle, repeated. They clinked glasses. "Thank you for being so patient with me, Chantelle. My mindfulness meditation practice made all the difference." Chantelle bowed her head, smiling. She sipped while Akar chugged, burped, and wiped his mouth with the back of his hand.

He looked around. "Where is everybody?" he asked. Chantelle's home was a well-orchestrated open floor plan perfect for fluid movement. But the guests had disappeared.

Chantelle nodded sideways, thick tresses tumbling around her shoulders and pulsing down her back. It was quite a change from the high bun she wore at work with tendrils framing her beautiful round face. Through the dining room was a ten-foot by ten-foot sunroom with glass walls. The sun streamed in, illuminating the room like a prism of light. Rashad, Brianna, and all the guests were happy as hot, sweaty, naked mole rats cuddling against each other.

"What's happening?" Akar asked in wonder.

"It happens every time I have people over. They all crowd in there." Chantelle cocked her head. In a dreamy voice she mused, "That's my meditation room. When I walk in there, I feel an immediate sense of peace and love. Maybe on some level, they feel it too."

The Takeaway

Mindfulness didn't make the CEO of Akar's company nicer. Nor did it cure Chantelle's husband's post-traumatic stress disorder caused by his military experiences. It wasn't a miracle cure, but it did allow Akar and Chantelle to weather challenges with much greater equanimity. It can do the same for you. Stay on your mindfulness journey. It will bring you greater peace.

WHERE YOU GO FROM HERE

Congratulations for completing *Mindful in 5,* the first book in this series! Consider revisiting chapters that challenged you. Some might take years to master, and that's perfectly all right because mindfulness is a journey, not a destination. Use this book as a reference tool to support you along your journey.

If you enjoyed taking this journey, please leave a review on Amazon. com if that's where you bought the book. If you bought it from spiwejefferson.com, please post your review at trustpilot.com and insert "Mindful in 5" for the company name. Use the QR code below to visit the website and download sample chapters for upcoming books, watch videos, check out podcast episodes, and sign up for companion emails, insider notices for upcoming books and events, and exclusive invitations to live meditations with Spiwe Jefferson.

Look for future titles in this series, including the companion journal for this book, the *God-Lovers Edition* and *Mindful in 5 for Busy Professionals.*

Now that you have tools to increase inner happiness starting with just five minutes a day, I sincerely hope you enjoy the benefits and harness the power of mindfulness to live and work to your highest and best purpose each day. Be mindful and be well.

Printed in the United States
by Baker & Taylor Publisher Services